Reducing your waistline

Dr Scott Chambers

Dr David Haslam

Reducing your waistline
First published – December 2006

Published by
CSF Medical Communications Ltd
1 Bankside, Lodge Road, Long Hanborough
Oxfordshire, OX29 8LJ, UK
T +44 (0)1993 885370 F +44 (0)1993 881868
enquiries@thesimpleguides.com
www.thesimpleguides.com

We are always interested in hearing from anyone
who has anything to add to our Simple Guides.
Please send your comments to *editor@thesimpleguides.com*.

Author Dr Scott Chambers
Medical Editor Dr David Haslam
Science Editor Dr Scott Chambers
Production Manager Emma Catherall
Layout Jamie McCansh and Julie Smith
Operations Manager Julia Savory
Publisher Stephen I'Anson

© CSF Medical Communications Ltd 2006

ISBN-10: 1-905466-27-7
ISBN-13: 978-190546-627-6

Printed in Great Britain.

Contents

INTRODUCTION

DR DAVID HASLAM

Clinical Director, National Obesity Forum

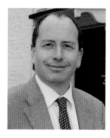 As a nation, we are getting fatter! Evidence of this can be seen all around us, from news coverage on an almost daily basis to voyeuristic 'entertainment' shows such as *Celebrity Fit Club*.

The UK has one of the fastest growing weight problems in the world. In the last quarter of a century alone, rates of obesity and overweight have virtually quadrupled. More worryingly, the obesity problem appears to be spiralling out of control. But the UK is not alone in having a problem; most of the world, including parts of the developing world, is in the midst of an epidemic of obesity and obesity-related ill health. The rise of this epidemic has been so rapid that many experts predict that obesity will soon overtake smoking as the number one preventable cause of death. The obesity 'time bomb' exploded long ago; we are now waiting for the almost inevitable diabetes, heart disease and premature death 'time bombs' to go off.

One major concern is the massive increase in obesity and overweight in children. This has the potential to cause a whole host of health problems for the next generation of adults. Indeed, it is a real and alarming possibility that the current generation of children may have a shorter life-expectancy than their parents if the obesity problem continues unabated. The gravity of the situation has been recognised by the UK government, which has set itself the improbable target of halting the year-on-year rise in childhood obesity by 2010.

Numerous explanations have been suggested for the recent explosion in obesity rates. Most of these focus on substantial changes that have occurred in our environment over the past three to four decades. One common sense explanation is that technological innovation has led to us become increasingly inactive in our daily work and leisure lives. Coupled with a wider access to energy-rich convenience food with a high fat, sugar and salt content, available on every street corner at any time of day or night, it is little wonder that we are getting fat! No longer do we need to hunt and gather scarce supplies of food and expend huge amounts of energy in the process. We can now literally drive up to the entrance of our out-of-town supermarkets and 'forage' amongst the array of attractively packaged processed foods on display. Put simply, we live in an environment that almost guarantees that we will get fat – a toxic, 'obesogenic' environment.

Most of us are aware that carrying too much weight is not good for our health. However, few of us appreciate that weight gain in itself is only part of the problem. Where excess fat is distributed in the body has a more important impact on our health. In particular, people who gain weight around their 'bellies' giving them a characteristic 'apple' shape (something the experts describe as 'abdominal', 'central' or 'visceral' obesity) have a much higher risk of developing serious life-threatening diseases such as type 2 diabetes and cardiovascular disease. These people often need support to reduce their waistlines in order to reduce this risk.

Despite increasing awareness of the health risks associated with being overweight or obese, many people find it a huge challenge to lose weight and achieve a healthy body shape. It's also a real challenge to keep that extra weight off in the long run. This is because weight loss requires us to make substantial changes to our 'normal' behaviour and requires motivation and perseverance for success. It's certainly not helped by living in an environment that actively encourages weight gain! As most overweight people will have gained their extra weight over the course of many years, it is important to recognise that it will take time to lose unhealthy weight and reduce those bulging waistlines.

It's not all bad news though! The loss of relatively modest amounts of weight can have a really positive impact on a person's health and quality of life. For example, the loss of about 5–10% of body weight, equates to a reduction of the dangerous fat within the abdomen by about 30% with a knock-on positive effect on other risk factors for serious disease such as cholesterol levels and blood pressure. Small amounts of weight loss will also help maintain motivation to continue with a weight-loss programme over the longer term.

Throughout this book, we will highlight some of the key issues associated with carrying extra weight, particularly around the waist. We will explore the lifestyle changes that you will need to adopt to reduce your risk of weight-related ill health, which will also serve to improve your general physical and mental health and well-being. We will also discuss some of the evidence-based treatments and other interventions that are effective for weight loss.

Specifically, this Simple Guide will answer the following questions.

- What is a healthy weight and how is it measured?
- What is a 'normal' body shape and how can an individual tell whether they are 'normal'?
- What is obesity and overweight?
- What causes obesity and overweight?
- What are the health risks of obesity and overweight?
- Why is extra fat stored around the abdomen such a health risk?
- What health benefits can an individual expect from losing weight?
- What lifestyle changes should be made to aid weight loss?
- What happens if weight loss attempts by lifestyle changes fail?
- What drugs or other measures are available that may help weight loss and reduce the risk of serious disease?
- How is the government addressing the problem of obesity?

By being more aware of these issues and by providing you with answers to these questions, you and your family will be armed with the information you need to achieve the body shape and healthier lifestyle that all of us desire.

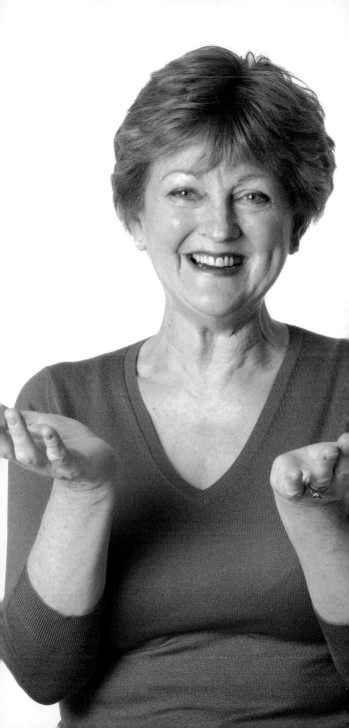

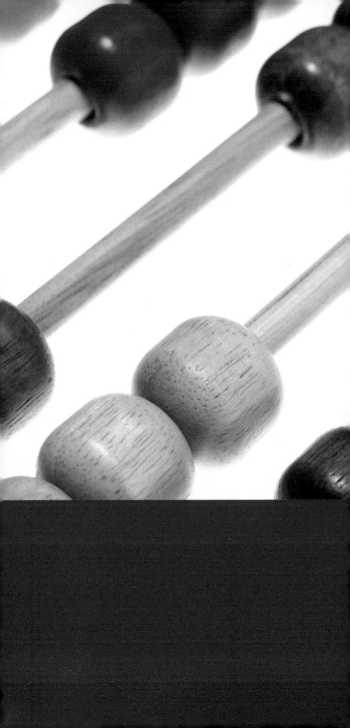

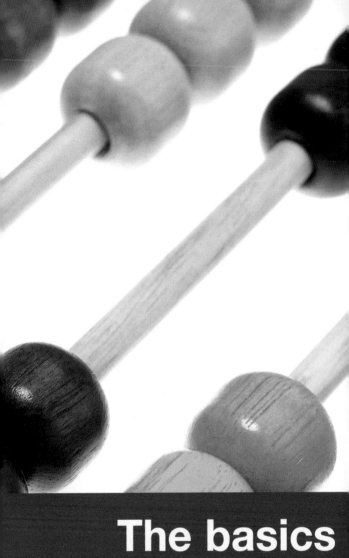

The basics

THE BASICS

Weight gain usually occurs over a long period of time as a result of an imbalance between the amount of energy consumed in your diet and the amount of energy expended during activity. You can shed inches from your waistline by becoming more active and by reducing the amount of calories that you consume; the so-called 'energy balance equation'.

WHAT IS OBESITY?

Obesity is defined as the accumulation of excessive amounts of body fat to such an extent that it can potentially cause serious health problems. Weight gain usually occurs over a long period of time due to an imbalance between the amount of energy consumed in the diet and the amount of energy expended during physical activity. By reversing this imbalance in favour of more energy expenditure and less energy intake, weight loss and improved health can be achieved.

In reality, obesity is a more complex disease and its development is influenced by environmental, genetic, social and cultural factors, many of which unfortunately lie beyond our control to change.

WHAT IS A HEALTHY WEIGHT?

The study of body weight and body shape is called 'anthropometry'. Several anthropometric

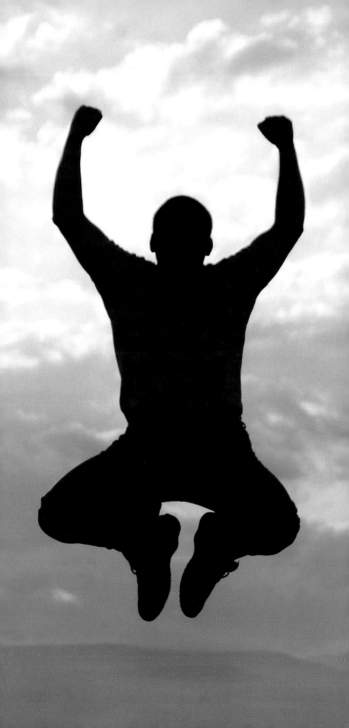

techniques are used by healthcare professionals to determine whether you are carrying too much weight which may be putting your health at risk.

Remember that you can also use these techniques to monitor your progress once you have begun a weight-loss programme. By observing changes in your body weight and body shape, it should help you to remain motivated to continue on your journey to a slimmer and healthier you!

Body Mass Index (BMI)

The **BMI** is probably the best known method of testing whether you are overweight. It requires a relatively straightforward calculation that you can perform in your own home. Simply follow the steps on the page opposite.

In general, a high BMI indicates that you are carrying too much fat which is putting you at an increased risk of weight-related disease such as diabetes and cardiovascular disease. A BMI above 25 is considered overweight whilst if you have a BMI above 30 you are considered to be clinically obese. Please don't be too alarmed by this label – it's a term doctors use to describe your weight and risk of ill health rather than a description of how you look. If your BMI is anywhere above 25, unless you have an athletic build, you really should consider losing weight. The tips for weight loss found later in this book will help you. Remember that you can make a real difference to your health from relatively modest weight loss.

CALCULATING YOUR BMI

It is relatively straightforward to calculate your BMI, to see whether you are overweight and at an increased risk of diabetes, cardiovascular disease and other health problems.

Grab a tape measure, a set of bathroom scales and a calculator and follow these simple steps:

(1) Measure your height in metres. Multiply this number by itself and write down the answer.

(2) Measure your weight in kilograms. Divide it by the number you wrote down in the first step.

(3) **The number you get is your BMI.**

Look on the chart below to see what your BMI means.

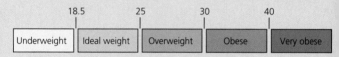

Remember that your BMI is only a broad indicator of your risk of ill health. Your risk is determined by your body shape. People with a very muscular build tend to have a higher BMI, but may not be unhealthily fat. On the other hand, some inactive individuals may have a low BMI but will be at a high risk because they carry large amounts of fat around their waist. Your age and gender will also affect your BMI. Men will have a slightly higher BMI before they are at risk of ill health because they are usually more muscular than women. However, it is best to stick to the guidelines above – they are the internationally accepted boundaries for both genders. Certain ethnic groups (e.g. South Asians) have an increased risk of ill health at a much lower BMI. Therefore, lower BMI thresholds apply in these populations.

This scale does not apply to children. However, age- and gender-specific BMI charts (adjusted for growth) are available to determine BMI in children.

You can also calculate your BMI online at *www.thesimpleguides.com*.

Waist circumference – a measure of body shape

Although the BMI is still widely used, it doesn't show where in your body the excess fat is stored. Measuring your waist circumference is a simpler tool which can tell you how much extra fat is accumulating in and around your abdomen. In addition, waist circumference is an accurate measure of health risk, is more easily measured than BMI (requiring only a tape measure and no calculation) and is a tangible figure, stated in inches or centimetres, rather than an abstract number, such as a BMI of 30.

Extra fat within and around your waist substantially increases your risk of a host of 'risk factors' including insulin resistance (a stage in the development of diabetes), high blood pressure and abnormal cholesterol levels and various diseases such as type 2 diabetes and cardiovascular disease. Consequently, waist circumference is probably a more useful measure for predicting complications of excess weight gain than the BMI alone.

As discussed previously, certain ethnic groups are at higher risk of weight-related illness at a much lower BMI. The same also

Insulin is the hormone manufactured by the pancreas that controls blood sugar levels and allows the tissues to utilise glucose as a fuel for basic biological processes.

A risk factor is something that increases your odds of developing a disease. Having multiple cardiovascular risk factors substantially increases your risk of cardiovascular disease.

applies for waist circumference, and so lower cut-offs for waist size have also been established for the Asian population compared with Europeans.

Remember that your waist circumference is not just the waist size of your trousers or skirt! Just because you can squeeze into an old pair of 38-inch jeans, it doesn't mean that your waist is not putting you at risk of ill health! To measure your waist circumference accurately, you will need to measure the distance around your middle at a point midway between the bottom of your ribs and the top of your hips at the side, keeping the tape measure parallel to the ground. Then check against the table overleaf to see if you are overweight.

If your waist circumference indicates that you are carrying an unhealthy amount of fat around your middle, you really need to take action by changing certain aspects of your lifestyle such as your diet and your current level of physical activity. To monitor your progress during any weight-management programme, always remember to measure the same site each time. As a general rule, by losing 1 kg in weight you should lose about 1 cm from your waistline.

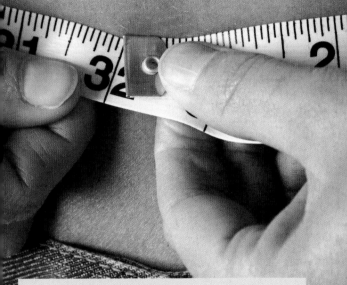

Measuring waist circumference

1   Take off your shirt and loosen your belt.

2   Position the tape mid-way between the top pf
    your hip bones and the bottom of your rib cage.

3   When taking measurement, the abdomen should
    be relaxed and you should be breathing out.

4   Record the measurement.

5   Check against the table opposite to see if your
    waistline is putting you at risk of ill health.

	Increased risk of disease	High risk of disease
European men	94 cm (or 37 inches)	102 cm (or 40 inches)
Asian men	–	90 cm (or 36 inches)
European women	80 cm (or 32 inches)	88 cm (or 35 inches)
Asian women	–	80 cm (or 32 inches)

Waist-to-hip ratio

This can be calculated by dividing your waist circumference by your hip circumference. A large study – the INTERHEART study – has shown that the waist-to-hip ratio is a valuable tool to determine your risk of obesity-related disease and, in particular, heart attacks (see *Why me?* page 38). INTERHEART showed that more than 90% of heart attacks in the world are avoidable and that a reduction in obesity is one of the most important measures a person can take to reduce their risk. Carrying extra weight around your waist increases your health risk more than carrying extra weight around the hips, thighs or buttocks. In fact, a large hip circumference appears to reduce your risk of diabetes and heart disease. For men, a waist-to-hip ratio of 1.0 or higher is considered to increase your risk of adverse health consequences. For women, the corresponding ratio is 0.9 or higher.

Other measures of body weight and shape

Technological devices such as body fat analysers are becoming increasingly popular and can be purchased relatively inexpensively from a variety of retail outlets. They measure the total amount of fat in your body and can be a useful additional tool to help you monitor your health improvements as a result of change in lifestyle. Although these devices may augment traditional measures such as waist circumference or BMI, for simplicity most doctors would recommend that you follow your progress by simply measuring your waist and weight.

More recently, CT and MRI scans have been used to more accurately map the distribution of body fat. However, these scans are expensive and equipment is scarce. In addition, they involve exposing patients to X-rays and so their use for repeated measurements is limited, and they have no place in routine weight management.

WHAT IS AN UNHEALTHY BODY SHAPE?

You may have heard people describe body shape in different ways. People who carry extra fat around their waists are often described as having an 'apple shape' whereas those who carry extra weight on their hips and buttocks are said to be 'pear-shaped'. Overweight women are traditionally pear-shaped, whilst overweight men are more likely to be apple-shaped, though some overweight women can also be apple-shaped, particularly after the menopause. Measuring your waist circumference will show you whether you are an apple or a pear. As we have already seen, there is a much greater concern about fat that is located around the abdomen and apple-shaped people have an increased risk of a variety of serious conditions including heart disease, strokes and diabetes.

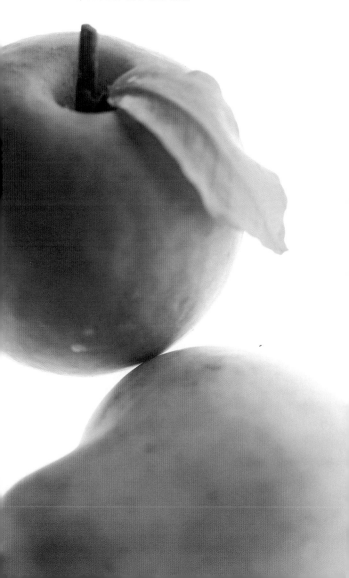

WHY IS ABDOMINAL FAT SO BAD?

Many vital organs lie within the abdominal cavity including your liver and pancreas. The excess risk associated with abdominal fat relates to the accumulation of fat around and within these organs, particularly the liver. The liver plays an important role in various metabolic processes in the body including the control of glucose and cholesterol levels, and its function can be altered substantially in the presence of too much fat. In addition, the fat itself can be considered as an organ in its own right as it secretes a variety of biologically active molecules that directly alter how the body responds to insulin and how it controls the metabolism of cholesterol, amongst other functions. This is discussed in more detail in *Simple science* (page 60).

WHAT CAUSES OBESITY AND OVERWEIGHT?

The reasons why people gain weight are diverse but essentially relate to an imbalance in how much energy is taken in as food and how much energy is expended during activity. However, there are a number of other factors that may increase your chances of becoming overweight that we should consider here. For example, there are a number of medical conditions that can make you put on weight.

MEDICAL CAUSES OF OBESITY

Endocrine (hormonal) problems

- Cushing's syndrome
- Disorders such as heart failure (these disorders cause fluid retention rather than true obesity)
- Thyroid disease (hypothyroidism – under active thyroid gland)
- Sex hormone changes (including hyperandrogenism)
- Growth hormone deficiency
- Rare chromosomal abnormalities that are diagnosed in childhood

Psychiatric problems

- Depression and eating disorders such as Binge Eating Disorder and Night Eating Syndrome

In addition, a variety of commonly prescribed drugs are also associated with weight gain. Your doctor may have told you if one of the drugs he or she prescribes increases your risk of weight gain. If you are worried that you are putting too much weight on, don't hesitate to discuss it with your doctor at the earliest opportunity. However, remember that these drugs are prescribed for a reason, and it is likely that the benefits you get from taking them over the longer term will outweigh the risks of the weight you gain in the short term. You can always use some of the techniques described throughout this book to help you lose some of the extra weight you gain whilst on treatment.

PRESCRIPTION DRUGS ASSOCIATED WITH WEIGHT GAIN

- Antidiabetic drugs (e.g. sulphonylureas, glitazones and insulin)
- Anticonvulsant drugs (e.g. sodium valproate, gabapentin, vigabatrin)
- Antidepressants (e.g. tricyclic antidepressants, mirtazapine, lithium)
- Antihistamines
- Antipsychotic drugs (e.g. olanzapine, risperidone)
- Corticosteroids
- The contraceptive pill and hormone replacement therapy (HRT)
- Beta-blockers
- Pizotifen

Genetics

A number of studies have shown a strong link between our genes and the development of obesity. Studies of identical twins brought up by adoptive parents have shown that the BMI of the twins was more similar to the BMI of their biological parents than to that of the adoptive parents. Although obesity and weight problems do appear to run in families, it is likely that many different genes are involved and these are likely to interact in a complex fashion with various environmental factors to exert their 'obesogenic' effects.

There are, however, a number of very rare genetic diseases that are associated with obesity. These include disorders such as the

Prader–Willi and the Bardet–Biedl syndromes. In addition, some individuals have a genetic defect in the gene that produces a hormone called leptin, which is involved in appetite control. You can read more about leptin in *Simple science* (page 56).

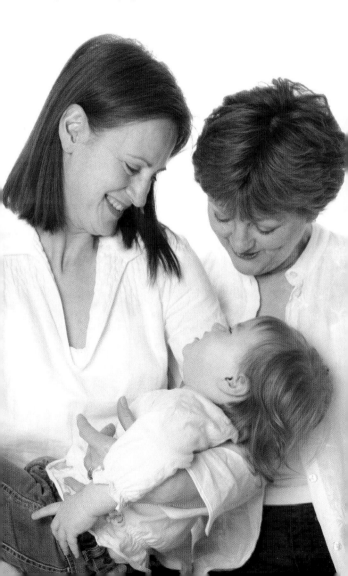

WHAT ARE THE HEALTH RISKS OF OBESITY?

Many aspects of your physical and mental health are affected by your weight and body shape. Indeed, it has been known throughout history that obesity is a cause of serious ill health and a lower life expectancy. Obesity and overweight can increase your blood pressure and your cholesterol levels and alter your body's response to insulin and glucose, all of which are associated with an increased risk of coronary heart disease, strokes and type 2 diabetes. It can also lead to pain, discomfort and unhappiness.

The figure opposite highlights some of the major health concerns associated with carrying excess weight, particularly around the abdomen.

However, there is good news! By losing relatively modest amounts of weight by adopting a more active lifestyle and a healthy, balanced diet, you will be taking great strides towards a healthier and better you! Unfortunately, the longer you remain overweight, the more damage you will be doing to your health in the longer term. So if you are overweight, remember don't delay those changes to your lifestyle and start feeling the benefits straight away.

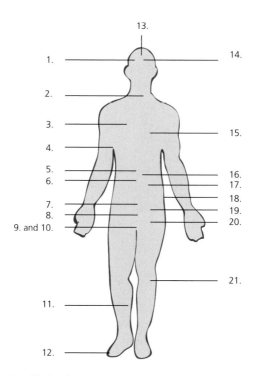

1. Eyes (blindness)
2. Windpipe + lungs (breathlessness, sleep apnoea, snoring, worsening of asthma)
3. Breast (cancer)
4. Armpits (sweating)
5. Stomach (digestive complaints, cancer)
6. Gallbladder (gallstones, cancer)
7. Bladder (urinary incontinence)
8. Pancreas (type 2 diabetes)
9. Women: uterus, cervix (complications during pregnancy, cancer)
10. Men: penis + prostate gland (impotence, cancer)
11. Legs (varicose veins)
12. Gout
13. Mind (low self-esteem, depression, eating disorders)
14. Brain (stroke from high blood pressure, Alzheimer's disease)
15. Heart (coronary heart disease from abnormal cholesterol levels, heart failure, enlargement, erratic beat, other types of heart disease)
16. Liver (liver disease)
17. Kidneys (stones, kidney failure from high blood pressure)
18. Back (lower back pain)
19. Colon + rectum (cancer)
20. Women: ovaries (reduced fertility, polycystic ovary syndrome, cancer)
21. Joints (arthritis, particularly of the knee)

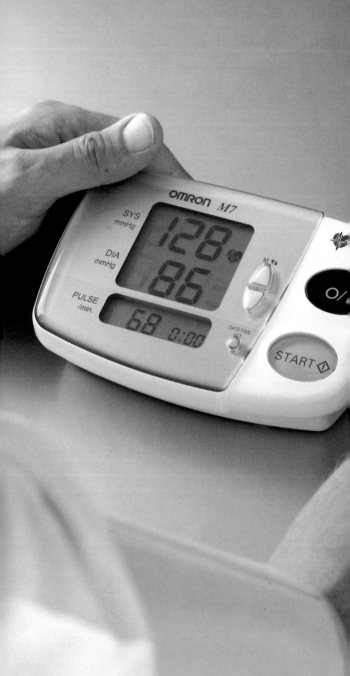

WHAT ELSE WILL MY GP CHECK?

Your GP will want to take a full history including when and why you think you have gained weight, and what methods (successful or otherwise) you have used to try and combat the problem. He or she will make a note of your ethnicity and will also want to know which members of your family have suffered from weight problems, and whether or not they also had diseases linked to obesity. If you have had problems with blood pressure or blood sugar levels during pregnancy, or if you have a family history of illness, you may be at increased risk. The medications you currently take are important, as are your smoking, drinking, eating and activity habits, which can be easily recorded in a diary. Your doctor or nurse will probably ask about any current symptoms such as chest pain, or excess thirst and urination in case you already have an obesity-related illness which has not been diagnosed.

As obesity and overweight are associated with so many different health problems and risk factors your doctor will also carry out a thorough check on your general health. He or she may take blood samples to test your cholesterol and glucose levels and to see if your thyroid gland is functioning as it should. They will also want to check your blood pressure and may book you in for an ECG to check that your heart is working properly. Other tests such as urine tests and chest X-rays will also be done at your doctor's discretion, depending on the findings of the other tests.

From these tests, they will be able to calculate your risk of a future heart attack or stroke, something doctors call your 'cardiovascular risk'. To help them work this out, your doctor will also ask you some questions such as:

- are you a smoker and if so how much do you smoke?

- are you a drinker and if so how much alcohol do you drink?

- is there a history of high blood pressure in your family?

- have you or anyone in your family ever suffered with any heart problems or diabetes?

- do you engage in regular exercise?

Your cardiovascular risk is an indication of the likelihood that you will have a heart attack or suffer a stroke, usually specified as a percentage over a period of 10 years. Cardiovascular risk is calculated to determine whether preventative drug treatment is required to reduce your risk (e.g. blood pressure-lowering drugs, cholesterol-lowering drugs, aspirin). Try calculating your own cardiovascular risk with our calculator online at *www.thesimpleguides.com* and consider seeing your doctor or nurse if the result is raised.

Risk factors for cardiovascular disease and type 2 diabetes appear to cluster in people with obesity and weight problems. This observation has led experts to come up with the concept of the 'metabolic syndrome', a collective term used to describe the clustering of different risk factors in individual patients preceding the development of cardiovascular disease and type 2 diabetes. Abdominal obesity lies at the core of this syndrome (see *Why me?* page 42).

REDUCING YOUR WAISTLINE

Weight loss is difficult to achieve and to maintain in the long run, and should never be underestimated. By setting yourself achievable goals, having realistic expectations and maintaining a positive attitude, you can expect to be successful in losing weight and shedding some inches from your waistline.

Set realistic goals

Most people will have gained weight over many months and years. So it is important to accept that it will take you some time to lose that extra weight. You will need to persevere to be successful, but remember, even relatively modest weight loss can significantly improve your health.

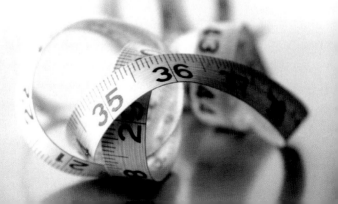

Lifestyle changes

By adopting a healthy, balanced diet and becoming more physically active, you can go a long way to losing some of your extra weight and improving your physical and mental health. Some people may need professional support to help them make these changes, and your GP or nurse may be an appropriate first port of call in this regard. Sharing your experiences of weight loss with others in support groups and slimming groups such as Weight Watchers may also help you to maintain motivation in order for you to achieve sufficient weight loss and keep those extra pounds off once you have lost them.

We will explore different ideas for a healthier lifestyle in the final section of the book. But in the meantime, here are some quick recommendations.

GENERAL RECOMMENDATIONS FOR A HEALTHIER LIFESTYLE

(1) Increase physical activity to a minimum of 30 minutes of moderate-to-vigorous activity each day to maintain current health. However, 60–90 minutes is recommended to lose weight and to keep the weight you have lost off.

(2) Reduce the amount of calories that you eat in your diet.

(3) Quit smoking.

(4) Reduce your salt intake.

(5) If you do drink, make sure it is within the recommended limits.

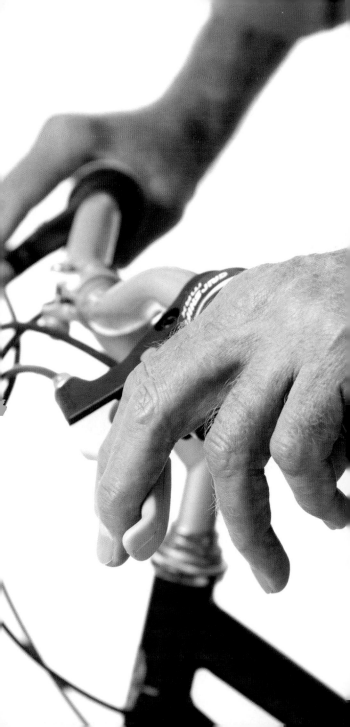

Long-term weight maintenance

An important aspect of any weight-loss programme is the need to keep the extra weight off once you have lost it. Sadly, many people who have successfully lost weight pile on the pounds again afterwards because they think that they can go back to living the same lifestyle as they did before. It is important to remember that any lifestyle changes that you make really need to be **lifelong**. This may sound daunting, but by making a few healthier lifestyle choices you will begin to feel better physically and mentally, which should encourage you to continue in the long run. Evidence suggests that keeping physically active is particularly important for long-term weight maintenance. Remember, by keeping fit your general health will benefit too.

Drug therapy

If you have made a serious attempt to lose weight by making changes to your diet and by becoming more active, but yet you remain overweight and at risk of weight-related ill health, your doctor may consider prescribing you a drug to help you lose a few more pounds. Your doctor will discuss with you the potential benefits and limitations of drug therapy including any untoward side-effects that may occur. It is important to remember that it is vital to continue with your new lifestyle whilst taking these drugs for them to be as effective as possible.

Three drugs are widely used in the UK to assist a weight-loss programme:

- orlistat (Xenical®)
- sibutramine (Reductil®)
- rimonabant (Acomplia®).

Each of these drugs has substantial evidence showing their effectiveness when used in combination with diet and exercise, and can allow patients to lose up to 10% or more of their body weight. More information about each of these drugs can be found in *Reducing your waistline* (page 92).

Other drugs such as phentermine and ionamin are very occasionally prescribed to certain patients. However, the evidence supporting their use is distinctly lacking and consequently they have no place in the long term management of obesity and are best avoided.

Surgery

Surgical options for obesity are currently reserved as an intervention of last resort for people who are morbidly obese and who are in need of immediate weight loss to reduce their heightened risk of ill health. As with any surgical intervention, there is an inherent risk from the anaesthetic and complications from the procedure. Unfortunately, this risk is increased in people who are obese. People who are eligible for surgery require extensive assessment prior to the operation and also require long-term monitoring afterwards.

Managing other risk factors

In addition to addressing your weight problem, your doctor will treat other risk factors that you will probably have as a result of the extra weight you are carrying. He or she may need to prescribe you drugs to reduce your risk from problems such as high blood pressure, abnormal cholesterol levels and high blood glucose. Don't worry though. These drugs have to go through rigorous checks on their safety and effectiveness. By losing weight and keeping these risk factors in check, you will be substantially reducing your risk of cardiovascular disease and type 2 diabetes.

BENEFITS OF 10% WEIGHT LOSS

1   A fall in premature death by about 20–25%.

2   A fall in diabetes-related death of about 30%.

3   A fall in obesity-related cancers by about 40%.

4   A fall in blood pressure of about 10/20 mmHg.

5   A fall of 50% in the risk of developing diabetes.

6   A fall in glucose levels of about 30–50%.

7   A fall in total cholesterol of about 10%.

8   A fall in LDL cholesterol (bad cholesterol) of about 15%.

9   A fall in triglycerides of about 30%.

10 A rise in protective HDL cholesterol of about 8%.

Sleep apnoea is a condition in which the affected individual stops breathing for short periods of time during their sleep. Many people will have daytime sleepiness leading to inappropriate sleeping, sometimes behind the wheel of a car, lorry or bus, with potentially disastrous consequences.

Benefits from weight loss

If you successfully lose weight your entire physical and mental health and general well-being stands to benefit. Even by losing relatively modest amounts of weight and reducing your waist circumference by a few centimetres your can bring about really positive changes to your health. Just look at the box opposite and see what can be achieved.

Other benefits from weight loss include:

- a reduced risk of serious, life-threatening cancers
- improved fertility for women
- improved sexual performance for men
- less breathlessness, snoring and sleep apnoea
- less joint pain and better joint function
- improved mental health
- better fitting clothes.

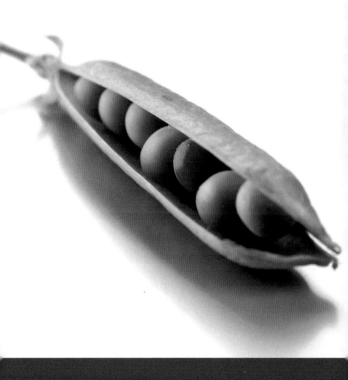

Why me?

WHY ME?

If you, or a member of your family, have a problem with your weight, then you are certainly not alone. Overweight and obesity and their associated health risks are such enormous problems that they have reached epidemic proportions throughout the world.

HOW COMMON IS OBESITY AND OVERWEIGHT?

The UK and much of the developed world is in the midst of an uncontrolled epidemic of obesity and obesity-related chronic (long-term) ill health. Across the world, it is estimated that about 1.1 billion people are overweight with about 312 million considered to be clinically obese. If we consider that lower thresholds for overweight and obesity apply in certain ethnic populations such as people from the Indian subcontinent, then the number of overweight people is probably closer to 1.7 billion. The problem has continued to rise over the past three decades and is continuing to increase to such an extent that many countries are considering obesity to be a serious public health crisis that requires urgent and radical action to resolve.

Between 1980 and 1997, obesity rates in England more than trebled from 6% to more than 20%. Today in the UK obesity affects about one-fifth of all men and a quarter of all women with more than 50% of the population believed to be overweight. On the basis of

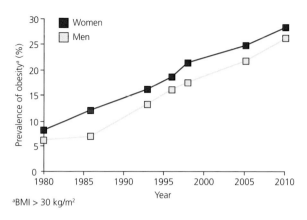

ᵃBMI > 30 kg/m²

TRENDS IN OBESITY PREVALENCE IN MEN AND WOMEN IN ENGLAND TO 2010.

current trends, it has been estimated that, by 2010, up to a quarter of all adults will be obese.

The UK has one of the biggest obesity problems in Europe. However, it is the USA that leads the world's obesity 'league table' with more than one-third of adults being clinically obese. This increases to up to 50% in certain ethnic groups. As the UK's rate of growth in obesity has mirrored that seen in the early years of the US epidemic, we can probably look to the USA to provide us with a snapshot of what we can expect to see in the future. If we don't take action now, we could expect a similar public health crisis here within the next 10 years. Indeed, experts predict that if no action is taken as much as three-quarters of the population can expect to be suffering the ill effects of excess weight within 15 years.

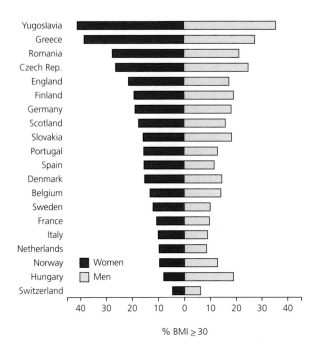

Yugoslavia
Greece
Romania
Czech Rep.
England
Finland
Germany
Scotland
Slovakia
Portugal
Spain
Denmark
Belgium
Sweden
France
Italy
Netherlands
Norway — Women
Hungary — Men
Switzerland

40 30 20 10 0 10 20 30 40

% BMI $\geq$ 30

OBESITY RATES IN SELECTED EUROPEAN COUNTRIES.

Perhaps somewhat surprisingly, the developing world is also experiencing an increase in obesity. This trend has gone hand in hand with increased wealth in these regions coupled with greater access to energy-dense food. Indeed, across the world there are now more over-nourished than malnourished people.

HOW COMMON IS ABDOMINAL OBESITY?

As we have seen, excess fat stored around the abdomen is a particular health problem and a strong predictor of weight-related ill health and premature death. In the UK, estimates suggest that about 29% of men and 26% of women have waistlines that are putting them at an increased risk of diseases such as cardiovascular disease and diabetes, both of which are associated with premature mortality. The problem is even more extreme in the USA, where more than half of all women have waists exceeding 88 cm (35 inches) and about a third of men having a waist above 102 cm (40 inches).

OBESITY IN CHILDHOOD

More than 80 million children and adolescents across Europe are now overweight or obese, with the UK again leading the way.

In the UK, childhood overweight and obesity has trebled since the 1980s, with about 10% of 6 year olds and 17% of 15 year olds now considered to be obese.

Although childhood obesity is a huge problem, the majority of the medical and economic burden of obesity arises in adulthood. Nevertheless, carrying excessive weight in childhood can lead to bullying, low self-esteem, social isolation and depression, factors which can perpetuate inactivity and comfort eating, exacerbating the weight problem further. Type 2 diabetes – traditionally an illness of middle and old age – is now being diagnosed in children and adolescents. Obesity also leads to respiratory and joint problems in kids. Obesity in childhood will also increase the chances that the child will enter adulthood with a host of health problems, whilst obese children are also more likely to become obese adults. As bad eating habits are formed early in life they are more difficult to change, such that a child that is exposed to a poor diet is more likely to have a poor diet as an adult. This is why it is so important to act now to halt the continued progression of the problem in childhood.

Certain risk factors appear to have an impact on obesity early in life. For example, watching more than 4 hours of TV each day has been shown to increase the likelihood of childhood obesity. There is also growing evidence that sleep deprivation, particularly in childhood, is associated with weight gain (see *Simple science,* page 58). Finally, if mothers smoke during pregnancy, the child's risk of obesity also increases.

Your child's chances of becoming overweight or obese may have been predetermined before they were even born. There is increasing interest amongst scientists in the link between conditions in the womb during foetal development and the development of obesity. This is something the experts called 'intrauterine programming'. Both under-nutrition and over-nutrition during foetal development appears to increase the risk of overweight and obesity and lead to alterations

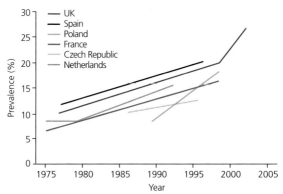

More than 80 million European children and adolescents are now overweight and obese.

CHILDHOOD OBESITY IN SELECTED EUROPEAN COUNTRIES.

in metabolism and insulin sensitivity. In addition, patterns of growth after a child is born also appear to be very important. A low weight at birth followed by a rapid and excessive weight gain beyond the age of 1, appears to be a particularly strong risk factor for obesity and increases the risk of cardiovascular disease and type 2 diabetes in later life.

Breast-feeding is believed to protect against obesity in later life for both the mother and the child. Breast-fed babies naturally start to consume less milk after about 8 weeks, and will naturally fall onto a lower growth curve. Remember, that this is quite normal. 'Topping up' the baby to maintain its original growth pattern is potentially dangerous, and may induce childhood obesity.

THE BURDEN OF OBESITY-RELATED ILL HEALTH

Although the massive increase in the obesity problem in the UK is set to impose a legacy of serious ill health on future generations, we are already seeing its adverse effects. For example, type 2 diabetes, previously a disease of middle age, is now manifesting in increasingly younger children as a direct result of the obesity epidemic. In fact, in many areas of the UK, there are now more cases of type 2 diabetes in children than there are of juvenile (type 1) diabetes.

The World Health Organization estimates that more than 115 million people in the world are living with ill health associated with obesity. It has been predicted that obesity and its associated diseases will soon overtake infectious disease as the biggest killer across the globe. In the UK, it has been estimated that about 30,000 premature deaths occur each year (about 6% of all deaths) as a direct result of obesity, with an average reduction in life expectancy of about 9 years. If there were 1 million fewer obese people in the UK, there would be about 15,000 fewer cases of coronary heart disease, 34,000 fewer cases of type 2 diabetes and 99,000 fewer people with high blood pressure.

Cardiovascular disease

Diseases of the heart and the blood vessels – collectively called cardiovascular disease – account for about 40% of all the deaths in the UK and represent the biggest cause of death in our country. Coronary heart disease accounts for about half of these deaths, making it the most important form of cardiovascular disease. In addition, heart disease accounts for 22% and 13% of all premature deaths amongst men and women, respectively.

Obesity, and particularly abdominal obesity, is an important risk factor for the development of cardiovascular disease. People with a high BMI (BMI >29) have a four-fold increased risk of coronary heart disease compared with those whose BMI is normal. In addition, type 2 diabetes (another consequence of obesity) is a major risk factor for the development of cardiovascular disease, with approximately three-quarters of deaths amongst people with diabetes being attributed to cardiovascular disease.

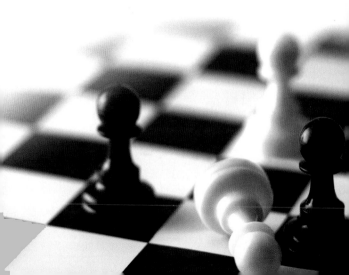

The INTERHEART study

INTERHEART was one of the largest investigations into the worldwide incidence of heart disease ever conducted and gathered information from 52 countries including more than 15,000 people who had previously suffered a heart attack.

INTERHEART identified nine risk factors that accounted for the vast majority of these heart attacks. These risk factors included: smoking, abnormal lipid levels, high blood pressure, diabetes, abdominal obesity and certain psychosocial factors. Factors that were protective against heart attacks include diet, physical activity and moderate alcohol consumption.

There was a particularly strong association between abdominal obesity and the risk of heart attack, with about one-third of heart attacks linked to excessive weight around the abdomen.

Type 2 diabetes

Type 2 diabetes is one of the word's most common chronic diseases. Like obesity, diabetes has reached epidemic proportions in the developed world and continues to increase dramatically in the developing world. Indeed, the epidemic of diabetes mirrors the epidemic of obesity, which neatly highlights the close link between the two, and has prompted experts to coin the term diabesity to describe this connection.

Globally, about 200 million people have diabetes, with about three-quarters of these cases being type 2 diabetes. This number is expected to rise by more than one-third to 370 million by

2030. In the UK, the prevalence of diabetes is expected to rise from a reported 1.8 million cases in 2000 to more than 2.5 million by 2030. However, this is probably an underestimate because as many as 1 million cases are thought to be undiagnosed.

More than 80% of people with type 2 diabetes are overweight or obese and it is widely believed that excess weight is the main factor that contributes to the development of the disease in these people. Women who are in the highest BMI group (BMI above 35) have a more than 90-fold increased risk of type 2 diabetes compared with those whose BMI is normal (under 22).

But why does being overweight cause type 2 diabetes? Excess fat and excess fat around the abdomen in particular reduces the sensitivity of the cells to insulin. This 'insulin resistance' is an important stage in the development of type 2 diabetes and is associated with a variety of additional metabolic problems, including the development of abnormal cholesterol levels, high blood pressure and high blood glucose levels. About a quarter of the UK population are thought to have insulin resistance without being aware of it.

Type 2 diabetes is itself associated with a range of serious diseases and complications including eye disease, kidney disease, coronary heart disease and strokes. The longer you have type 2 diabetes, the higher your risk will be of developing these complications. If your blood sugar level, and hence your diabetes, is poorly controlled, these complications can begin to occur at an earlier age.

High blood pressure

Obesity and overweight are major factors underpinning the rapidly increasing incidence of high blood pressure (or hypertension) in the world. It is now thought that about 1 billion people worldwide have high blood pressure.

In general, the heavier you get, the higher your blood pressure climbs. For example, the average systolic blood pressure (that's the top number in your blood pressure reading) is about six units higher in obese people compared with those of a normal healthy weight. Obese people appear to have about a five-times higher risk of hypertension than people of normal weight and up to two-thirds of all cases of 'essential' hypertension (high blood pressure without a definite medical cause) are found in people whose BMI exceeds 25.

But why does increased body weight increase blood pressure? There are a number of plausible explanations. First, an increase in weight requires an increase in the volume of blood to feed the tissues. Second, the blood of overweight people is generally more viscous and sticky. Third, fat cells (adipocytes) in the abdominal region secrete substances that constrict blood vessels and directly increase blood pressure. Finally, a diet which promotes obesity usually has high levels of sugar and saturated fat and may also contain large quantities of salt, which is known to be a leading cause of hypertension.

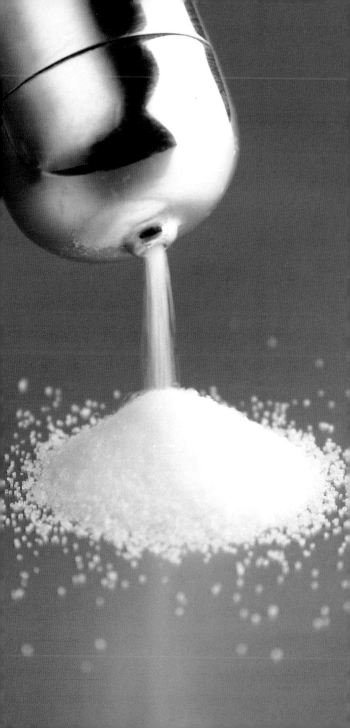

High cholesterol

About two-thirds of the population have cholesterol levels higher than 5 mmol/L. The most recent guidelines in the UK recommend that the total cholesterol level should not exceed 4 mmol/L. This means that many people in this country are living with a cholesterol level that is putting them at an increased risk of cardiovascular disease and premature mortality.

If you are overweight or obese, you are more likely to have higher cholesterol levels compared with a person of normal weight. In addition, if you have a large waistline, it is highly likely that the balance of different types of cholesterol and other 'lipids' will have become disturbed, something called dyslipidaemia. This means that you will have low levels of a protective type of cholesterol (HDL cholesterol), and high levels of two bad types of lipid, LDL cholesterol and triglycerides.

The metabolic syndrome

The metabolic syndrome is a collective term used to describe the clustering of a number of risk factors that precede cardiovascular disease, type 2 diabetes and certain cancers. These risk factors include abdominal obesity, high blood pressure, high blood lipid levels and high insulin levels. High insulin levels – technically called hyperinsulinaemia – develop as a direct result of

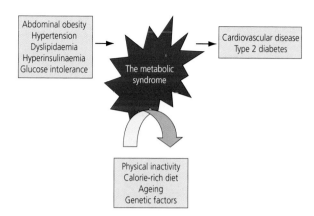

THE METABOLIC SYNDROME.

insulin resistance; the pancreas attempts to overcome the insensitivity of tissues to insulin by increasing its production. Abdominal obesity and insulin resistance appear to be the core features of the metabolic syndrome. If you have the metabolic syndrome, you are at increased risk of developing type 2 diabetes, as well as a range of other conditions such as heart disease and stroke. The metabolic syndrome currently affects about one quarter of the UK population.

WHY HAVE I BECOME OVERWEIGHT?

There are many reasons why you may have gained weight, but the main reason is that your energy balance has become disrupted in such a way that you are not expending enough energy during physical activity for the amount of calories that you are consuming in your diet. This could be because you are leading a particularly hectic lifestyle that makes it difficult for you to cook meals from fresh natural ingredients or you may be finding it difficult to find the time to fit in enough physical activity. Your personal circumstances may also have changed. For example, you may have given up smoking, moved in with a partner or you may have given birth, all of which are associated with weight gain. Taking on a new job or retirement can also lead to changes to a normal eating routine and activity levels with a knock-on effect on weight.

There are a number of other risk factors that may predispose you to weight gain. These include:

- having a parent who is overweight or obese
- being female
- getting older
- coming from a certain ethnic group (e.g. South Asian or Afro Caribbean)
- mental health problems such as depression
- learning disabilities.

Excess weight also appears to be linked to socioeconomic status and whereabouts you live in the country. For, example, obesity is more common in Scotland and Wales than in England. Regions with high social deprivation generally have higher rates of obesity compared with wealthier areas. Excess weight is also linked to your occupation, with unskilled manual workers being more likely to be overweight. Again, you are more likely to be overweight if your family income level is in the low range, compared with higher earners.

WHAT FACTORS ARE RESPONSIBLE FOR THE OBESITY EPIDEMIC?

The epidemic of obesity reflects substantial changes that have occurred in our environment over the past few decades. As we saw in *The basics*, obesity arises from an imbalance between energy expenditure and energy intake. Increasingly sedentary lifestyles coupled with poor diets have become the norm in recent decades and appear to be responsible for the obesity problem and the epidemic of associated ill health.

Changes to our diet

Our diet, how and where we eat and our general relationship with food have all changed substantially in recent years. Nowadays, we are surrounded night and day by tempting convenience food from fast food restaurants and supermarkets which is high in fat, sugar and salt, and of course calories! These foods are heavily promoted to consumers by advertisers and food retailers, and are available at a lower real cost than ever before. In addition, portion sizes have shot up in recent years, particularly since the advent of the 'super-size' option in fast food outlets; the quality of ingredients has also deteriorated whilst fast food is available on every street corner at all times of day and night. Children in particular seem to be most at risk from these practices. Cartoon characters and celebrity endorsement of certain unhealthy foods undoubtedly increase the appeal of such foods to children, and may in part explain the rapidly increasing problem of obesity in childhood in the UK.

Whilst our fat consumption has shot up in the latter part of the twentieth century, the carbohydrate content of our diets has fallen

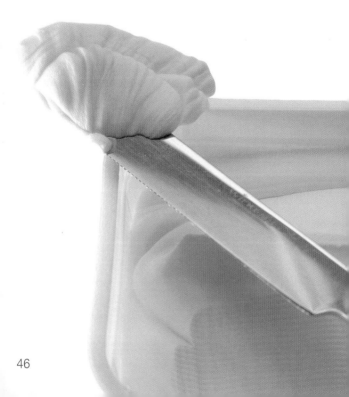

primarily because we are cooking less from scratch with fresh natural ingredients. Given that fat in the diet yields more calories of energy than carbohydrate, it is hardly surprising that our nation has got fatter, particularly now we are less active and not as able to burn off the excess energy!

It has been estimated that, on average, adults in the UK eat about 20 calories more each day than they expend during physical activity. Over the course of a year, this excess calorific intake equates to a 1 kg increase in weight. Over a 10-year period this relative small excess intake would lead to a gain in weight of about one and a half stone!

The box below summarises some of the key changes to our diet and our relationship with food that have occurred in recent years.

1   Increased consumption of fast food.

2   Increased availability of highly processed foods packed full of fat, sugar and salt.

3   Larger portion sizes.

4   More snacking and grazing.

5   Inaccurate food labelling.

6   Intensive advertising and promotion.

Physical inactivity

Early humans required huge amounts of energy to allow them to hunt and gather food. Fat was laid down during periods of plenty to provide an energy store to supply energy needs during periods of famine. Therefore, there was a survival advantage for those who laid down more fat. However, nowadays food is in such plentiful supply and so rich in calories that our sedentary lifestyles make it much harder to burn this extra energy. The extra fat we lay down as a consequence has become a major disadvantage!

It has been estimated that about 40% of women and 30% of men are considered to be inactive in the UK. Many people do not engage in exercise as they get older and are less exposed to organised sporting activities than they would have been at school or university.

Five reasons for inactivity in adult life

1   Increased urbanisation.

2   Increase in the use of the car, train or bus rather than walking.

3   Less active, office-bound jobs.

4   Increased leisure time in the pub or in front of the TV or PC.

5   Out-of-town shopping centres with large car parks.

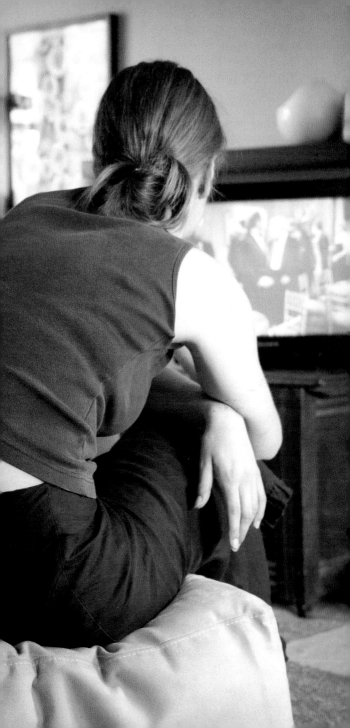

Five reasons for inactivity in childhood

1   Many children no longer walk to school.

2   Too many hours spent in front of the TV and computer.

3   Less time spent on organised school sports.

4   Playing fields have been sold off.

5   Increased safety concerns.

Opportunities for physical activity amongst children have become more limited in recent years due to a number of reasons, and it is now estimated that about 30% of boys and 40% of girls are insufficiently active. Children are playing more video games than ball games and are watching more TV. Many schools no longer partake in competitive sports and others have even sold off their playing fields to property developers!

Many experts believe that it is the inactivity side of the 'energy equation' that has driven the obesity epidemic, with changes to diet only having a relatively recent impact on the upward trend in obesity prevalence.

Affluence

At one time, being fat was seen to be an advantage during times of famine and was often seen as a sign of wealth. Increasing relative wealth during the twentieth century may have allowed people greater access to energy-dense food coupled with the ability to purchase technological labour-saving devices that have reduced physical activity.

A good example of the relationship between wealth and obesity is illustrated by the island of Naura. This small Pacific Island experienced a rapid increase in its economic wealth when guano deposits – phosphate-rich bird droppings useful for fertiliser – were discovered. The population became more wealthy almost overnight and with it obesity took hold. Prior to this new-found wealth, type 2 diabetes did not exist to any appreciable extent. Now about 30% of the population of the island have the condition and it is the most common cause of death.

THE SOCIOECONOMIC IMPACT OF OBESITY AND OVERWEIGHT

The obesity epidemic in the UK is already having a huge financial impact on the NHS and the economy. Some experts believe that if the obesity problem isn't tackled urgently then it may even have the potential to bankrupt the health service in the future!

Each year, obesity and its related illness are thought to cost the UK economy about £3.5 billion. Cardiovascular disease, for which obesity is a major risk factor, costs even more – about £30 billion. About 18 million working days are lost each year due to obesity-related sickness. Thus, effective weight control for the whole population has the potential to provide socioeconomic as well as health benefits.

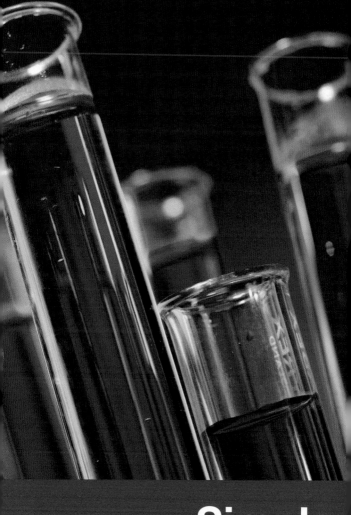

Simple
science

SIMPLE SCIENCE

The human body has a variety of sophisticated mechanisms that control your hunger and appetite. When these systems fail, overeating can occur causing you to gain weight. Drugs that influence these and other processes have an important role to play in weight management.

WHY DOES YOUR BODY NEED FOOD?

Food provides a source of energy for every activity that your body performs, from moving and keeping warm to internal biological processes that we aren't consciously aware of. Different people need different amounts of energy depending on how active they are. In general, the more active you are, the more energy you will need.

Normally, your brain helps to keep your weight in check by issuing a series of 'signals' that balance how much you eat and how much energy is burned by the cells of your body. These signals come in the form of hunger to stimulate eating, or satiety (or fullness) to stop you eating. In some obese and overweight people these signals do not seem to work properly.

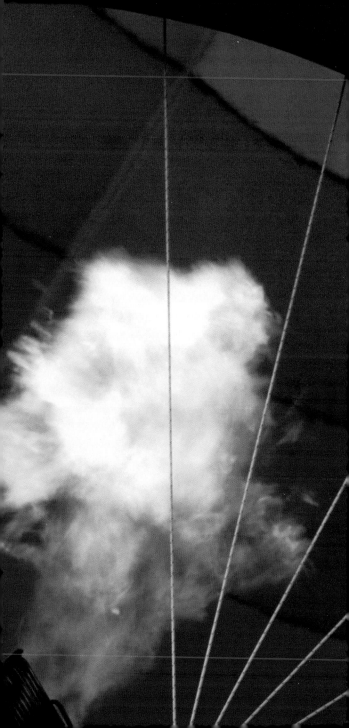

CONTROL OF APPETITE – THE ROLE OF HUNGER HORMONES

Scientific and medical research has led to the identification of two key 'hunger hormones' – leptin and ghrelin – that are involved in controlling our eating behaviour.

Leptin is synthesised and secreted from adipose tissue in direct proportion to the amount of fat stored in the body. Therefore, leptin can be considered as a kind of messenger that provides the brain with information on total fat stores. If the amount of fat falls, for example during starvation, then levels of leptin fall and, via a series of complex signalling events, the brain is stimulated to encourage food intake and reduce energy expenditure thereby increasing weight. Some individuals with weight problems appear to have a problem with how leptin works, though this seems to occur very infrequently. In some people, the gene that produces leptin is faulty and consequently they do not produce enough of the hormone. As a consequence, hunger is stimulated and overeating and obesity may occur. Other overweight people appear to have built up a resistance over time to the appetite-suppressing effects of leptin, possibly as a result of failure of the brain to recognise the leptin signal. So, leptin levels remain high but the brain does not appear to respond in the appropriate fashion.

Ghrelin appears to have the opposite effect to leptin. When it is present at high levels it stimulates appetite, fat production and growth, leading to an increase in food intake and body weight. It is secreted by the stomach in response to food intake, but is also synthesised in a number of other tissues, including the kidney, the pituitary gland and hypothalamus of the brain. Ghrelin also stimulates the release of growth hormone in the brain which also stimulates feeding and weight gain.

The hypothalamus is a key region of the brain that is intimately involved in the control of appetite.

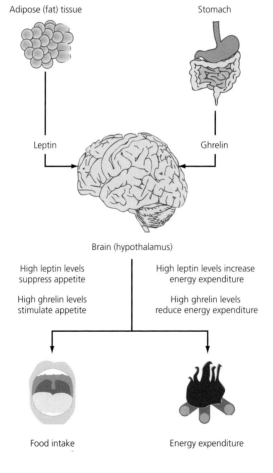

Adipose (fat) tissue

Stomach

Leptin

Ghrelin

Brain (hypothalamus)

High leptin levels suppress appetite

High leptin levels increase energy expenditure

High ghrelin levels stimulate appetite

High ghrelin levels reduce energy expenditure

Food intake

Energy expenditure

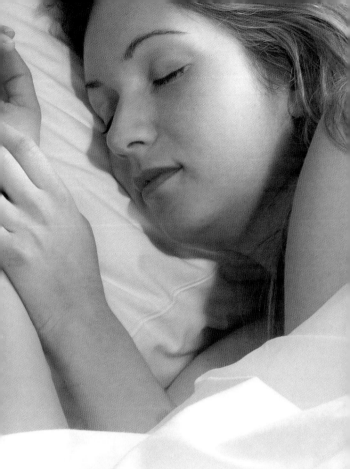

Hunger hormones and sleep

Recently, there has been growing interest in the link between obesity and sleep deprivation, particularly in childhood (see *Why me?* page 33). It is now known that shorter sleep times are associated with increased ghrelin levels and decreased leptin levels, the net effect of which is increased appetite and decreased energy expenditure and thus a propensity to put on weight. Although this research is in its infancy, it certainly could account for the possible link

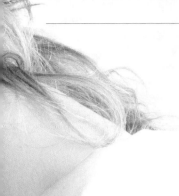

between reduced sleep and increased weight. Researchers have also shown that a diet rich in good carbohydrates (e.g. wholegrains) or high in protein suppresses ghrelin more effectively than a diet high in fat.

Serotonin

Within the brain, chemicals called neurotransmitters are involved in generating signals of hunger and satiety. One of the most important neurotransmitters is serotonin. It has been known for quite some time that abnormalities in the levels of this neurotransmitter may lead to overeating and the development of obesity. For example, it is known that increased activity of serotonin within the central nervous system is associated with the suppression of food intake. Likewise, low levels of this neurotransmitter may stimulate overeating. Consequently, a number of different drugs have been developed that have attempted to boost the serotonin signal in an effort to increase satiety. Some of these early drugs did indeed suppress appetite but unfortunately had some serious side-effects. Since then, however, research has continued and has led to the development of a newer drug that boosts the satiety signal and appears to be safer than the older generation drugs. This drug is called sibutramine and you can read more about this in *Reducing your waistline* (page 95).

WHAT IS THE ROLE OF FAT AND ABDOMINAL FAT?

For many years fat (or adipose tissue as it is technically known) was considered to be an inert storage depot that cushioned the body's organs, provided insulation and acted as a source of energy during periods of food shortage. Although fat certainly has these functions, it is now becoming increasingly recognised that adipose tissue is in fact a metabolically active organ that secretes a whole array of biologically active products including hormones and cytokines which influence many important biological processes, including how glucose and lipids such as cholesterol are metabolised. Some of these factors also appear to have an immune function.

The function of adipose tissue is also influenced by where in the body it is stored. As we have seen, when excess fat is stored within the abdomen it substantially increases the risk of the development of serious diseases such as coronary heart disease and type 2 diabetes. It is now thought that the increased risk associated with abdominally located fat arises from a difference in the synthesis of these biologically active products in this type of fat compared with fat that is located subcutaneously (under the skin). So, in the presence of excessive amounts of abdominal adipose tissue, more of the bioactive hormones and cytokines are produced. The net effect of this cascade of biological activity is an increase in the body's resistance to insulin, a disruption in the cholesterol profile and an increase in blood pressure. These observations therefore provide an explanation as to why excessive amounts of abdominal fat increase the risk of so many different 'cardiometabolic' disorders.

A cytokine is a small protein that has specific effects on how cells interact and communicate with one another. In this way, they influence various different biological processes. When a cytokine is secreted from adipose tissue it is called an adipocytokine.

ADIPONECTIN

Adiponectin is one of a group of substances (the adipocytokines) secreted by the metabolically active adipocytes that are located within the abdomen. Many of these substances, and adiponectin in particular, have been attracting interest from scientists because of their potential role in the development of obesity-related diseases. Other adipocytokines include resistin, tumour necrosis factor alpha and interleukin 6.

Abdominal obesity appears to be associated with low levels of adiponectin. In turn, it is thought that low adiponectin levels decrease the sensitivity of tissues to insulin (insulin resistance). In particular, as the liver does not respond to the insulin signal as a result of the low adiponectin levels, glucose production from the liver is not inhibited and blood glucose levels rise. This is a stage in the development of type 2 diabetes.

Low adiponectin levels are also thought to lead to a reduction in good HDL cholesterol levels and an increase in a particularly harmful form of LDL cholesterol.

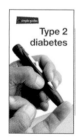

For more information see
Type 2 diabetes

In summary, adiponectin appears to underpin all of the risk factors associated with abdominal obesity. Current scientific research is looking at possible ways to increase adiponectin levels in an attempt to protect against obesity-related diseases.

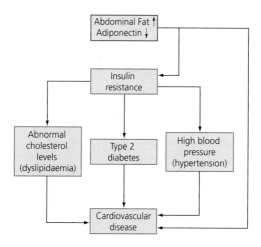

THE ENDOCANNABINOID SYSTEM

Researchers have recently discovered another important biological system that plays an important role in how our appetite is regulated in the brain. Interestingly, this system was discovered from studies into why cannabis users get 'the munchies' after smoking the drug. Chemicals in cannabis – called cannabinoids – bind to specific receptors in the brain which leads to a whole signalling cascade that stimulates a feeling of hunger. Obviously, eating is the natural response to quell this hunger.

Further work has shown that this system of signalling pathways in the brain remains overactive in overweight and obese people and in some other people who have addictive behaviours such as smokers and some drug users. Consequently, researchers came up with the idea that if the activity of the system can be inhibited in some way it would follow that it would reduce the urge to eat and hopefully reduce weight.

This idea led to the development of a new type of drug that specifically blocked the effects of the endocannabinoid system. This drug, called rimonabant (Acomplia®) was introduced onto the UK market in 2006. You can read more about rimonabant in *Reducing your waistline* (page 96).

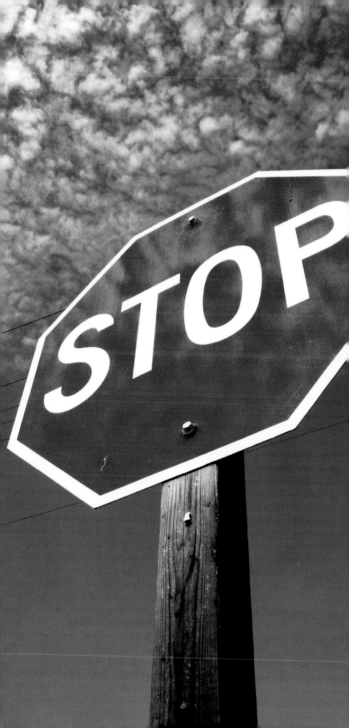

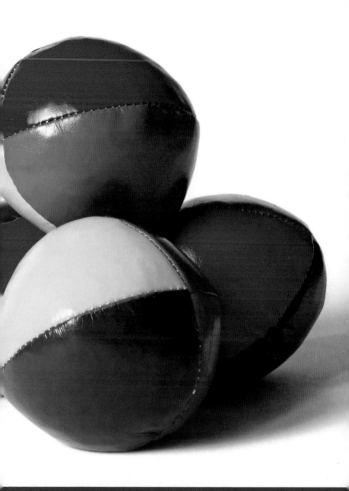

Reducing your
waistline

REDUCING YOUR WAISTLINE

In order to reduce the health risks associated with having a large waistline, it is important that you set yourself some realistic and achievable weight-loss goals. By working closely with your doctor and other members of your healthcare team, your chances of long-term success will improve.

WEIGHT AND WAIST MANAGEMENT

Losing weight and shedding inches from your waistline is all about eating fewer calories than you burn off in your everyday life. Therefore, the best way to tackle any weight problem is through a combination of a healthy balanced diet and regular physical activity.

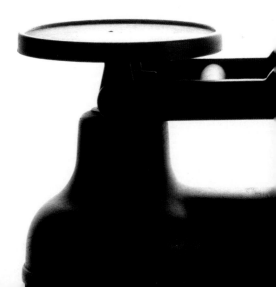

By losing weight, many aspects of your physical and mental health stand to benefit. But don't underestimate any weight-loss programme. It's very important to acknowledge and accept that weight loss isn't easy and that it requires some lifelong changes in your behaviour for long-term success. These changes will require the support of your family and friends, but also require a positive attitude from you. However, many people find that seeking help from their doctor or other health professional to tailor a weight-loss programme to their personal circumstances helps them to achieve their weight goals.

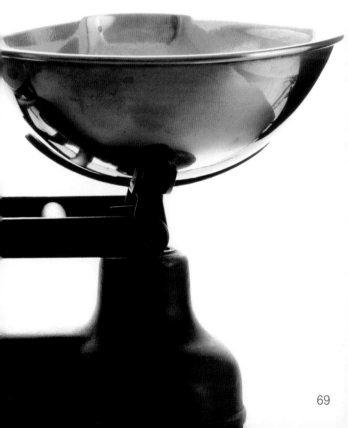

BEHAVIOURAL CHANGES

In order to be successful at losing weight, it's necessary to evaluate your current eating habits and your current level of physical activity before making the necessary long-term changes to behaviour. Like any habit, eating habits are often very difficult to change (particularly if they have been established in childhood), and this requires motivation, setting of realistic targets, confidence and positive attitude, flexibility and, more often than not, professional support.

Make a plan and set yourself achievable goals

You will not have gained weight overnight and chances are that your weight has crept up over many months and years without you really noticing. Although how you have lived your life over these years will have contributed to you being overweight or obese, you should not feel that you are solely to blame for your condition. It is very difficult for anyone to maintain a health body weight and body shape in an environment that actively encourages you to put on weight.

Given that your weight will have crept up over a long period, you certainly shouldn't expect any quick fixes to your weight problem. Any self-respecting weight-loss programme will not guarantee rapid weight loss, and most experts believe that you should be aiming for a slow and steady weight loss of about 0.5–1.0 kg per week (that's about 1–2 lbs) over a period of about 3–6 months. That way you will be far more successful at losing weight and keeping the extra weight off in the long run.

Scientific evidence suggests that the most striking benefits from weight loss appear to come from losing between 5 and 10% of your baseline weight, particularly when the excess weight is lost from your waist. Many studies have shown that this level of weight loss is associated with an improvement in a variety of health outcomes, including an increase in life expectancy of up to 4 years in people with type 2 diabetes. We have already looked at the benefits from this amount of weight loss in *The basics* (page 26).

Look at the table below so that you can see how much weight you should be aiming to lose.

Starting weight	5% weight loss is:	10% weight loss is:
70 kg (11 stone)	3.5 kg (8 lb)	7 kg (1 stone 2 lb)
89 kg (14 stone)	4.5 kg (10 lb)	9 kg (1 stone 6 lb)
102 kg (16 stone)	5 kg (11 lb)	10 kg (1 stone 8 lb)
115 kg (18 stone)	6 kg (13 lbs)	11.5 kg (1 stone 11 lb)
127 kg (20 stone)	6.5 kg (1 stone)	13 kg (2 stone)

How long should this weight loss take?

The table below provides a rough guide on the amount of time you can expect it to take you to lose a set amount of weight. Remember, to be effective in the long-term, weight loss should be slow and steady and should be at a rate of about 0.5–1.0 kg a week. Why not fill in the third column with your own personal target date based on this rate of weight loss.

Desired weight loss:	Range of time:	I will achieve this by:
3 kg (7 lb)	3–6 weeks	
6.5 kg (14 lb)	7–13 weeks	
13 kg (2 stone)	3–6 months	
19 kg (3 stone)	5–10 months	

'A journey of a thousand miles begins with a single step'

The best way to succeed with any of the lifestyle changes described in the subsequent sections of this book is to make small and steady changes to your life rather than being 'gung ho' and changing everything at once. Be realistic and you will have more chance of success at keeping the extra weight off in the longer term. Setting unrealistic and unachievable goals for weight loss will inevitably lead to disappointment. If you do have any lapses in your weight-loss programme, try not to be too disheartened. Try to use the experience positively so that you are able to deal with similar situations better in the future.

Food and activity diaries

Before you start any weight-loss programme, it is helpful to evaluate your starting position. Using food and activity diaries can help you and your doctor identify existing patterns of behaviour and will also help you to identify the triggers and situations that encourage you to eat too much and exercise too little.

Ask yourself questions such as what am I eating and why am I eating it? Be honest with your answers though. Many people genuinely believe they are eating far less than they actually do. A food diary (if you keep it up to date and are honest with yourself) will show you just how much you are eating and what triggers you to eat. By working with your GP or other members of the healthcare team, you can find ways of overcoming these triggers and then you can plan ways of overcoming them and any other barriers you may have to adopting a healthier lifestyle.

Monitoring

To stay motivated with anything in life, it is important that you see results! Weight loss is no exception. Keep an eye on how much you weigh and check your waist circumference each week. But don't do it every day. You will have small fluctuations in your weight on a daily basis and weighing yourself at the wrong time can give you an inaccurate picture and can be disheartening. You may also want to keep an eye on the results of blood tests that your doctor gives you. Seeing a positive effect on your cholesterol level or blood pressure can show you that your weight-loss programme is having a huge and positive effect on your life.

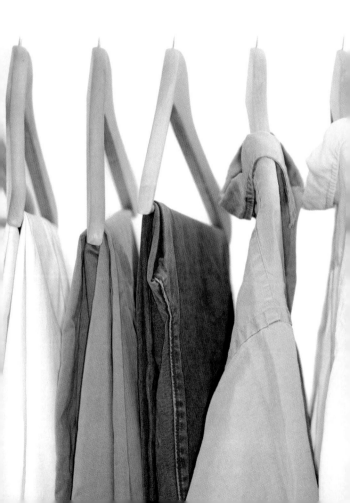

Rewards for success

Once you've set yourself some realistic goals
and you have committed to a weight-loss
programme, it is worth thinking about some
rewards that you can give to yourself if you
achieve your targets. This may give you an
incentive to work towards. However, remember
to make them healthy rewards! For example,
why not give yourself a beauty treatment, or
buy a new item of clothing or a CD or book.

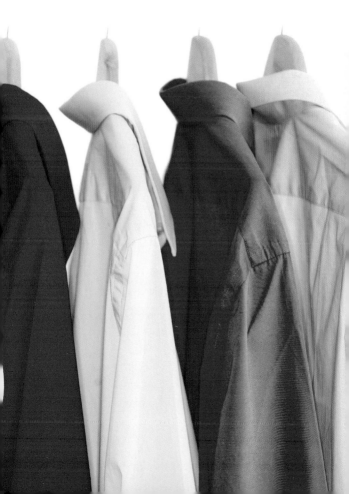

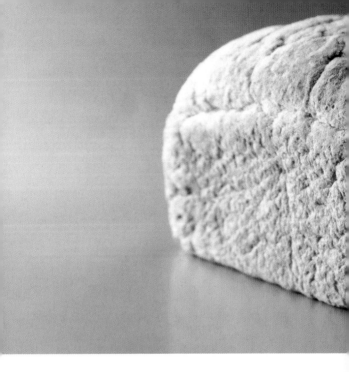

PRACTICAL ADVICE FOR LIFESTYLE CHANGE

Before you embark on any programme of weight loss, it is advisable to think honestly about your lifestyle and how you can best implement changes that will help you lose weight and improve your health.

1 Eat a healthy and balanced diet

Everybody can benefit from a healthy, well-balanced diet, not just those who are overweight or obese. By involving your family and friends and encouraging all of them to eat healthier, it will make things easier for you and better for them in the long run too.

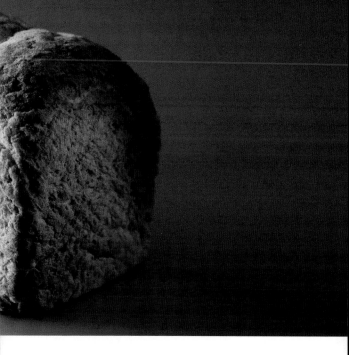

What is a healthy diet?

A healthy diet is one that:

■ is rich in fibre-containing starchy foods, such as wholemeal bread, pasta and rice, and cereals without any added sugar

■ is low in fat (particularly saturated fat), sugar and salt

■ is packed with fresh fruits and vegetables.

The government's Food Standards Agency (*www.food.gov.uk*) has produced a picture guide called *The Balance of Good Health*, which shows the proportions of the five main food groups (i.e. bread, cereals and potatoes; fruit and vegetables; milk and dairy products; meat, fish and alternatives; fatty and sugary foods)

THE BALANCE OF GOOD HEALTH

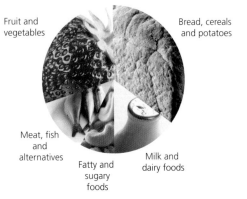

Fruit and
vegetables

Bread, cereals
and potatoes

Meat, fish
and
alternatives

Fatty and
sugary
foods

Milk and
dairy foods

that you should be aiming to eat each day. The
size of the section on the plate taken up by
each type of food represents what proportion
of your diet it should make up. However, it is
important to remember that *The Balance of
Good Health* is a guide to nutritional eating and
not a weight-loss diet in itself.

**TOP 10 TIPS FOR WEIGHT LOSS WITH A
HEALTHY DIET**

1 Try not to skip meals. Eat regularly to
avoid hunger pangs which make you
snack. Make sure you eat breakfast. Try a
bowl of cereal, a piece of fruit or a slice of
wholemeal toast.

2 Enjoy your food. Eating more slowly fills
you up more, so you won't feel the need
to eat as much. Use meal times as a time
for the whole family; eat around the
dinner table and enjoy their company – it's
amazing how much slower you eat than
when you eat in front of the TV!

3 Only eat when you are hungry and avoid snacking particularly on high-energy snacks like crisps and chocolate.

4 Watch your portion sizes but feel free to 'go large' on fruit and vegetables and other foods which are high in fibre as these will fill you up and satisfy your hunger.

5 Cut back on fat. Try low sugar versions of sugary foods and drinks. Use less salt.

6 Aim for variety – look out for low-calorie, low-fat recipes and try new things.

7 Change how you cook. Cook meals from scratch with fresh fruit and vegetables and steam, boil, bake, grill rather than fry!

8 Remember that alcohol contains more calories than you might expect.

9 Plan your meals and make a shopping list. Don't shop when you're hungry!

10 Weigh yourself and measure your waist once a week. If you weigh yourself more regularly you will only get disheartened by the ups and downs in your weight that occur naturally.

As we already discussed, you should aim to lose weight gradually, and following *The Balance of Good Health* model will help you to do this.

As well as eating the different food types in the correct proportions, it is also important that you don't eat too big a portion of food. Try using a smaller plate or smaller utensils and leave something on it when you have finished.

How much do I need to eat?

There are recommended guidelines for how many calories and how much fat you should be including in your daily diet. Although these limits depend on your level of physical activity, they do act as a useful guide. If you stick with these limits, you will maintain a healthy weight. However, if you need to lose weight, you will need to reduce the amount of calories in your diet and increase the amount of physical activity you engage in.

RECOMMENDED DAILY ALLOWANCES FOR THE AVERAGE ADULT

Each day	Women	Men
Calories	2000	2500
Fat	70 g (saturates 20 g)	95 g (saturates 30 g)

Most experts believe that you should be trying to aim to reduce your daily calorie intake by about 500–600 calories each day below the recommended daily intake for successful weight loss. By reducing your daily calorie intake by this amount you can expect to lose about 0.5 kg a week. That may not sound like an awful lot, but you'll be surprised how quickly it builds up and improves your health. Look at it another way. If you ate about 100 extra calories a day every day for a year, you could expect to put on about 4 kg (that's about 9 pounds). And remember, by losing weight slowly you'll reduce the chances of regaining it again later.

What about fat?

Although you are trying to lose weight, do not aim to eliminate fat altogether. Your diet needs to be balanced and a small amount of fat is vitally important to allow your body to function properly. For example, fats give structure to all the cells of your body and there are some vitamins that are only soluble in fat. It's all about choosing the right fats and using them to replace bad fats in your diet.

Aim to:

■ keep within your total recommended daily allowance of fats

■ replace saturated fat with polyunsaturated fats or monounsaturated fats

■ avoid 'trans' fats (look out for 'hydrogenated' or 'partially hydrogenated' fats and vegetable oils on food labels; this type of fat has been shown to be particularly harmful to our cardiovascular health).

Saturated animal fats and 'trans' fats increase the levels of lipids in your blood, including cholesterol and triglycerides. If you are overweight and have a high cholesterol level eating too much saturated fat and 'trans' fat will exacerbate this problem further. However, certain polyunsaturated fats on the other hand, do not have this effect on lipids. In fact, some of these fats actually improve the profile of lipids in your blood, increasing the amount of good cholesterol and reducing the amount of bad cholesterol. It is particularly important, therefore, to make sure that the majority of the fats that you eat are mono- or polyunsaturated.

Sources of unsaturated fats – good!	Sources of saturated fats – bad!
Oily fish	Fatty meat
Nuts and seeds	Cheese
Sunflower, olive and rapeseed oils and spreads	Lard, suet
Avocados	Cream
Olives	Cakes, pastries.

Commercial diets and slimming groups

Huge amounts of money are spent each year on a whole range of commercial diets, many of which proclaim miracle benefits in very short periods of time. However, many of these diets are best avoided, simply because rapid weight loss is not sustainable over the long-term. Another problem with commercial diets is that many of them lack the scientific evidence to give them any credence. However, there are some diets that do have a reasonable evidence base, which we will briefly touch upon below.

There are also a number of slimming groups in the UK that may be helpful if you require further help and support with your weight-loss programme. These include Weight Watchers, Rosemary Conley Diet and Fitness Clubs and Slimming World. In general, these programmes provide support through a weekly meeting and encourage healthy eating through structured food plans. Hearing other people's experiences of weight loss and individual success stories in these groups can be particularly useful in helping to motivate you to continue losing weight. However, these programmes require commitment and time, and can be expensive.

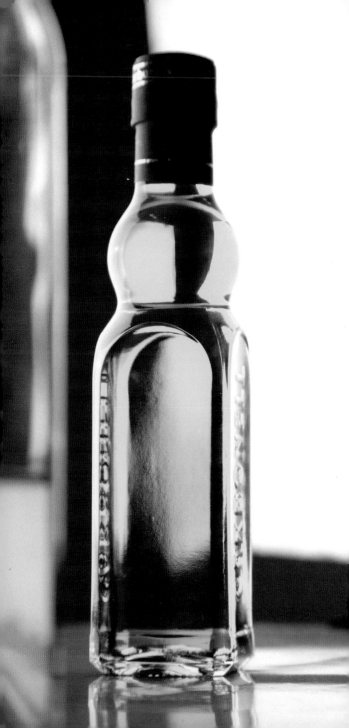

The 'low-carb' diet (e.g. the Atkins diet)

Nutritional guidelines recommend that you base your diet primarily on carbohydrates and proteins with a smaller contribution from fats. Controversially, some people believe that over-consumption of carbohydrates leads to weight gain and potentially obesity, type 2 diabetes and other health problems.

'Low-carb' diets involve a considerable restriction in the amount of carbohydrates in the diet. Instead, people on these diets eat an unrestricted amount of protein with additional calories obtained from fat. It may not seem a very sensible approach given the greater proportion of fat in the diet, but there is good evidence that this approach can help in weight-loss programmes, particularly for rapid weight loss in the short term, which may act as a useful starting point to motivate you to continue on your weight-loss journey. However, many experts are concerned that the Atkins diet may increase the risk of kidney damage and brittle bones and also increase already unhealthy cholesterol levels, although the accumulating evidence appears to suggests otherwise. You may also experience some side-effects from the diet such as headache, constipation, bad breath and fatigue.

Meal replacements

Meal replacements such as Slim-Fast are essentially low-energy products that are used to replace one or two meals each day. They usually come in the form of a drink like a milkshake or a cereal or chocolate snack bar. When used together with healthy eating advice they can help you stay on a low calorie diet and help you lose weight.

Other diets

For certain people, a very low-calorie diet may be appropriate. These diets severely restrict the number of calories you receive to under 800 a day. As you may not be getting enough vitamins and minerals with such a severely restricted diet, you may have to take appropriate supplements. Although there is plenty of evidence to show these extreme diets work, they are really only recommended for people whose weight is seriously threatening their immediate health, for example if they are having major breathing difficulties, or if they need to lose a lot of weight prior to obesity surgery.

THE BBC DIET TRIALS

Four diets have been evaluated in a large controlled trial as part of a BBC 'reality' TV programme called the *Diet Trials*. The four diets were: Slim-Fast, Weight Watchers, Atkins and Rosemary Conley. All four diets led to a significant weight loss averaging about 6 kg over 6 months, with no major differences between the groups. In the diets that used support groups (Weight Watchers and Rosemary Conley), the dieters were more likely to remain on the diet 12 months after starting the diet.

2 Get more physically active

By engaging in more physical activity you will be burning off extra calories and helping yourself lose weight. Remaining physically active will also help to keep the extra weight off in the long run. Try to involve your friends and your family in any activity that you chose – it will benefit them too, irrespective of whether or not they are overweight.

By becoming more active, you will not only help your weight but you will also benefit your health and well-being in many other ways. People who are more active often say that they have more energy, sleep better and feel great! Exercise has also been shown to reduce blood pressure, and cancer risk, improves the way the body handles glucose and also improves the balance of lipids in the blood. These benefits can potentially protect against coronary heart disease, strokes and type 2 diabetes. Exercise can also improve your general fitness, breathing problems, your mobility and bone health and can also alleviate stress and improve mental health.

Everyone can do something to increase their activity levels. You need not join a gym or take part in team sports. You don't even have to go out for a long run. Many activities that you undertake in your day-to-day life burn lots of energy. Just try to make sure you do more of them instead of sitting down for lengthy periods in front of the TV or computer! If you can, try cycling or walking to work rather than taking the car or bus. Get out in the garden and mow the lawn or hoover the carpets – they are great ways of burning calories too. Aerobic activity appears to be the best way of losing weight and it benefits cardiovascular health too! So aim to get a little bit breathless and a little bit sweaty! Exercises like brisk walking, dancing, cycling and swimming are ideal and can be great fun too, and organised exercise classes might be worth joining if you like to be around others who are in a similar situation.

TOP TIPS FOR BEING MORE ACTIVE

- Walk briskly for half-an-hour, five times a week.

- Choose stairs over lifts or escalators.

- Walk or cycle rather than using the car.

- Get out and about whenever possible – cut down on your time spent watching television or surfing the net!

- Encourage your family and friends to join you in a new active hobby – swimming or playing tennis, perhaps. Gyms often do special discounts for family membership.

Everybody should be aiming to exercise every day. The recommendation from the Department of Health is that all adults should be engaging in moderate to vigorous exercise for a minimum of 30 minutes a day on most days of the week. For children, the recommended amount is 60 minutes a day. This may sound daunting at first, and it may be that your current level of physical fitness will not allow you to partake to this extent. The key is to view this as a target. Start slowly and build up. You will soon notice changes in your fitness and stamina!

If you have been inactive for a long period of time it is vital that you build up any exercise plan slowly. Consider talking to your doctor first before you start exercising – they may be able to offer you further help and advice. In fact, GPs are increasingly able to refer patients to local gyms and sports centres where they can use the facilities for a reduced fee during off-peak times and also get support from exercise professionals. Why not ask your GP if such a scheme is operating in your area.

Pedometer

One way of keeping track of how active you have been is to use a pedometer. Many people are now using these little gadgets to keep track of their physical fitness and they are widely available in the shops. They simply fit around your belt and count how many steps you take during the day. The more steps you take, the more active you have been. Simple as that!

You should try and aim for a goal of 10,000 steps a day. But remember don't be too ambitious. Aim to build up the amount of steps you are taking over a few weeks until you reach this target, and then try to keep it at the 10,000 mark thereafter.

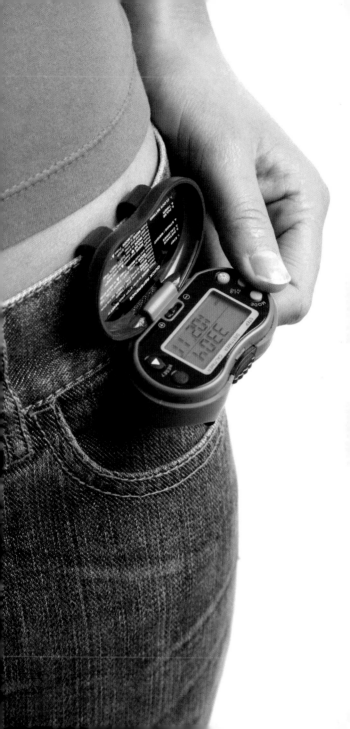

3 Reduce other lifestyle risk factors

Quit smoking

We all know that smoking is very dangerous and that it dramatically increases your chances of developing heart disease and having a stroke. We also know that it is associated with a wide range of cancers and some serious respiratory diseases.

Smoking is particularly dangerous if you are overweight or obese because you are already at a high risk of cardiovascular disease and other conditions compared with people who are of a healthy weight. If you smoke, your risk is increased even further. Your GP will be able to give you advice on how best to quit and will also be able to point you in the direction of other groups and helplines that you can contact for further support.

Remember that when you quit smoking you may unfortunately gain some weight. This happens because smoking appears to stimulate your metabolism, so that when you quit your metabolism slows down increasing the

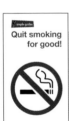

Quit smoking for good!

For more information see
Quit smoking for good!

likelihood of weight gain. Smoking also dulls your taste and smell which may also have a knock-on effect on your appetite. However, most experts would argue that it is far better for you to quit smoking straight away and address any weight gain afterwards rather than carry on smoking and put your health at very serious risk.

Drink alcohol in moderation

Increasing evidence suggests that moderate alcohol intake may actually be beneficial to our health, particularly our cardiovascular health. However, excessive consumption of alcohol is associated with liver disease, certain cancers, cardiomyopathy and accidents.

From the perspective of a weight-management programme, it is important to be aware that alcohol is a major source of energy and is very high in calories. As most people will know, alcohol also stimulates your appetite. Therefore, if you do drink, try to cut back. Aim to drink no more than two units of alcohol a day if you are a woman or three if you are a man, and try to have at least two alcohol-free days a week.

MAINTAINING WEIGHT LOSS

Sadly, despite their best efforts, many people will often put weight back on after losing it! But it doesn't have to be this way. By continuing with the changes that you have made to your lifestyle, you will be going a long way to keeping that weight off. Stick to a healthy eating plan and make sure you keep active. You may also want to keep monitoring your weight or waist, just to make sure it isn't creeping up again.

DRUG TREATMENT FOR OBESITY

If you have lost some weight by improving your diet and becoming more active, and yet you remain overweight and at risk of weigh-related ill health, or if you simply cannot lose weight by lifestyle changes alone, your doctor may consider prescribing you a drug to help you to lose more weight. Drug therapy can also help you to maintain the weight you have lost over the longer term. There are three drugs licensed in the UK for these purposes:

- orlistat (Xenical®)
- sibutramine (Reductil®)
- rimonabant (Acomplia®).

Historically, there has been some reluctance amongst doctors to prescribe drugs for weight loss. This reluctance stemmed from some problems with early generation drugs, including significant side-effects from amphetamine-based compounds and also from some serious complications which arose after using a particular combination of two drugs. However, there is plenty of evidence for the newer generation drugs that shows they are effective and well-tolerated even when used over the longer term.

You will take an active part in any decision to prescribe drug therapy. Your doctor will discuss with you the benefits and risks of drug treatment and will closely monitor your progress, keeping an eye on any untoward side-effects that may emerge. During treatment, your doctor will also want to monitor how much weight you are losing and may check your waist circumference to ensure that you are losing fat from your abdomen. They will also look to see if there any improvements in the physical signs of overweight such as immobility and breathing difficulties. Finally, they will also assess improvements in other cardiovascular risk factors such as your blood pressure, your blood glucose levels and your cholesterol profile.

In England and Wales, doctors follow guidelines issued by the National Institute for Health and Clinical Excellence (or NICE for short) when prescribing different drugs. NICE is an independent organisation that evaluates the clinical and cost-effectiveness of a variety of different treatments and other interventions on behalf of the NHS. NICE constantly reviews and updates its guidance and we would recommend that readers visit their website (*www.nice.org.uk*) for up-to-date information on what NICE has to say about the different drugs available.

In general, about two-thirds of patients will lose about 5–10% of their baseline body weight within 3–6 months of starting drug therapy but only if lifestyle changes continue. The manufacturers of all of these drugs provide excellent programmes of support that will assist you in maintaining a healthier lifestyle. Like any drug, it is vital that you remember to take your tablets as directed by your doctor, and you should also be aware that you will need to take your tablets for quite long time to avoid putting on weight that you have lost. You should be aware that you might put weight back on after you stop treatment, and so you should make every effort to continue with a healthy diet and remain active in the long run.

These drugs are not recommended for pregnant and breast-feeding women. They are also not yet licensed or recommended for children. However, very obese children at risk of ill health will be referred by your GP to a specialist who may consider surgery or off-label prescribing of these drugs.

Orlistat (Xenical®)

Orlistat is a novel drug that works by blocking the digestion of fat in the gut by inhibiting the enzyme involved in its breakdown. By doing so it stops the absorption of about one-third of the fat taken in the diet. Instead, fat passes out of your body into your stools. Given the high amount of energy in dietary fat, patients on orlistat can expect to see a reasonable reduction in body weight so long as they continue taking the drug. As orlistat is not absorbed into the body and is only active in the bowels it doesn't have the side-effects reported with earlier appetite-reducing medications. However, patients are encouraged to reduce the amount of fat in their diet as too much fat can cause a variety of unpleasant gastrointestinal effects. This, in part, may account for the effectiveness of orlistat in weight loss. Large clinical studies have also shown that orlistat also improves other cardiovascular risk factors including cholesterol levels and blood pressure, and can also significantly reduce the risk of developing diabetes. In patients already with diabetes, the weight loss achieved with orlistat helps to control blood sugar levels.

Sibutramine (Reductil®)

In contrast to orlistat, sibutramine is absorbed into the blood and works in a completely different way. It stimulates energy expenditure in the body and boosts signals from the brain that create a feeling of 'satiety' (pleasant feeling of fullness) thereby reducing the urge to eat. It achieves these effects by indirectly increasing the level of two chemical messengers (or neurotransmitters) in the hypothalamus of the brain. These neurotransmitters are called noradrenaline and serotonin. As sibutramine is absorbed into the blood stream, there are a number of rare side-effects from treatment that you should be aware of. These include headache, constipation, dry mouth, insomnia, nausea, light-headedness. Drinking more water may reduce these side-effects. Blood pressure can also increase with sibutramine therapy, and therefore your doctor will monitor your blood pressure before you start treatment and again throughout treatment, initially every fortnight. You may not be able to take sibutramine if you have uncontrolled high blood pressure or any other heart condition. Sibutramine should not be used for longer than 1 year.

Rimonabant (Acomplia®)

Rimonabant is licensed to help eligible patients lose weight in conjunction with a calorie-controlled diet. It works by blocking receptors in the brain called CB_1 (short for cannabinoid type-1) receptors. These form part of an important system that regulates appetite and thus body weight, and is also involved in other metabolic processes such as lipid and glucose metabolism. This system is called the endocannabinoid system or EC system and is described in more detail in *Simple science* (page 64).

The EC system is known to be over-activated in people who are overweight and obese and also in people with certain addictive behaviours such as smokers. Large clinical studies have shown that people who take rimonabant together with a programme of dietary change and increased physical activity show substantial weight loss over a period of up to 2 years. Not only do people lose weight, they lose fat from the right part of the body as shown by a substantial reduction in waist circumference in people receiving the drug.

Weight loss from rimonabant treatment improves a whole array of cardiometabolic risk factors such as blood cholesterol and glucose levels. In part, rimonabant appears to improve these risk factors independently of the weight loss that is achieved. This is because rimonabant appears to exert its effects not only in the brain where it suppresses appetite but also directly in fat tissue where it promotes the breakdown of fat and encourages adiponectin to be synthesised (see *Simple science,* page 62). Increases in adiponectin levels are known to improve the lipid profile and also to sensitise the cells of the body to the effects of insulin.

The safety profile of rimonabant appears to be good, though there have been reports of an increase in depression amongst users. Consequently, if your doctor prescribes you rimonabant he or she will monitor you closely through your treatment programme.

SURGERY FOR OBESITY (OR BARIATRIC SURGERY)

Bariatric surgery is currently only used as an option of last resort for people with severe morbid obesity who are in need of immediate weight loss to reduce their substantially increased risk of ill health. As with any surgical intervention, there is an inherent risk from the anaesthetic and complications from the procedure and this risk is increased in people who are obese. However, for many severely obese people, surgery can potentially be a life-saving intervention.

Patients being considered for surgery will be extensively assessed before surgery, will be given information, education and counselling about the potential risks and benefits of the procedures and will also be monitored closely for up to 18 months after the operation.

There are two basic types of surgery for obesity:

1 **Restrictive surgery.** Staples or inflatable bands are used to physically make the stomach smaller thereby creating a feeling of fullness with smaller portions of food. This type of surgery can be performed using a laparoscope (a thin fibre-optic cable), which reduces the risk for the patient compared with open surgery.

2 **Bypass surgery.** A more complex operation which involves connecting a small pouch from the stomach to the final segment of the small intestine, thereby bypassing a large part of the stomach and part of the small bowel. This obstructs the flow of nutrients and also reduces the opportunity for absorption of nutrients.

Bariatric surgery is highly effective and provides a permanent means of weight reduction. Weight loss can be dramatic and sustained, so much so that 90% of patients with type 2 diabetes no longer have the condition after surgery. Patients can eat a normal diet after the surgery, but in significantly smaller quantities.

Cosmetic interventions such as liposuction are not part of obesity management, because they do nothing to re-establish the energetic imbalance that characterises the obese and overweight state. In addition, as energy intake is unaffected, you are highly likely to put the weight back on again very quickly after the procedure. Finally, as liposuction removes fat located subcutaneously rather than the more dangerous fat localised around your abdomen, it does little to reduce your risk of weight-related ill health.

TREATING OTHER CARDIOVASCULAR RISK FACTORS

If you are overweight or are clinically obese, your doctor will need to address other risk factors that will increase your chances of long-term serious ill health. The lifestyle changes you are making to help you lose weight will help reduce the impact of these risk factors. However, if these risk factors are not controlled by the lifestyle changes that you have made, a

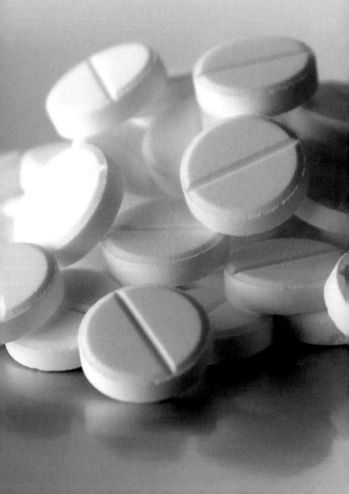

variety of drugs will be considered to help reduce your risk of complications such as type 2 diabetes and cardiovascular disease.

The following sections describe some of the drugs that lower raised blood pressure and cholesterol and improve how glucose is handled by the body. Your doctor may also give you drugs such as aspirin to thin your blood in an effort to reduce your cardiovascular risk.

Treatment of high blood pressure

Many overweight and obese people have high blood pressure. Therefore, your doctor will want to check your blood pressure at regular intervals and will treat your high blood pressure to ensure that it falls below 140/85 mmHg.

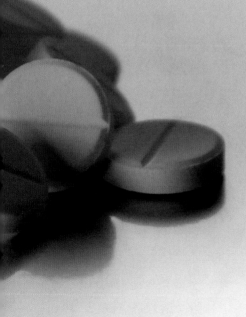

If you have diabetes, then you are considered to be at a much higher risk from the complications of high blood pressure and so your doctor will want you to achieve a lower target, which is currently set at 130/80 mmHg.

The lifestyle changes that you are making to help you lose weight will help to reduce your blood pressure if it is raised. However, if your blood pressure remains above the target level despite these changes, your doctor may prescribe you one or more of a range of blood pressure-lowering drugs.

As blood pressure can be difficult to bring under control, the chances are that you will need a combination of drugs from the range of different 'drug classes' available. Recent evidence suggests that newer types of blood pressure-lowering drugs such as the ACE inhibitors and angiotensin receptor blockers are more effective and safer than older generation drugs like beta-blockers and diuretics. In fact, beta-blockers may actually increase your risk of diabetes and are no longer routinely recommended for blood pressure control.

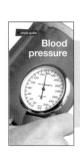

For more information see
Blood pressure

Treatment of high cholesterol

The higher your risk of cardiovascular disease, the more likely it is that your doctor will prescribe you medications to reduce your cholesterol. However, do remember that the lifestyle changes you are making to help you lose weight will also improve your cholesterol profile.

A number of different drugs are available to improve your cholesterol levels and they work in different ways. Some drugs are better at reducing LDL cholesterol (bad cholesterol) whilst others are better at lowering triglycerides and raising HDL cholesterol (good cholesterol). Statins are often the first choice of treatment because of the large amount of evidence that shows they work and are relatively safe. They are particularly effective at reducing LDL cholesterol. There is also evidence that statins can protect your heart in other ways. However, people with large waists often have low levels of HDL cholesterol and high levels of triglycerides yet their LDL cholesterol remains relatively normal. In these cases, your doctor may prescribe another drug such as nicotinic acid (although these drugs can be associated with some significant side-effects including hot flushes).

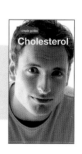

For more information see
Cholesterol

Treatment of type 2 diabetes

If you have type 2 diabetes some of the changes that you are making in your life to help you lose weight will also help you to control your blood sugar levels and may make your body more responsive to the effects of insulin. If you have diabetes, your doctor will monitor your blood sugar levels on a regular basis. If he or she finds that your blood sugar level is not adequately controlled despite the lifestyle changes that you have made, you may be prescribed antidiabetic tablets. Many patients with type 2 diabetes also often require insulin as well as drug therapy in order to control their blood sugar levels.

Unfortunately, treatment with some antidiabetic drugs actually increases people's weight and so your doctor will be very careful about selecting an appropriate drug for you. Sulphonylureas and insulin both cause significant weight increase, and both increase circulating insulin levels. There is evidence that the sulphonylureas in particular may cause the insulin-producing beta-cells of the pancreas to fail prematurely, thereby causing problems later in life. Metformin and drugs from the glitazone class of antidiabetic compounds appear to have a preferential mode of action. They work by increasing the body's sensitivity to the insulin that is already circulating in the bloodstream, which is beneficial for sugar control, the management of the other risk factors including cholesterol and blood pressure, and for the long-term benefit of patients. Glitazones are known to cause weight gain, but do so peripherally and not in the dangerous intra-abdominal region. Metformin can cause gastrointestinal upset and diarrhoea, but is now available in an inexpensive slow-release form which minimises these side-effects. In general, metformin is recommended first line for people who are overweight and require blood glucose control. Finally, antiobesity tablets such as sibutramine, orlistat and rimonabant are also helpful at reducing the risk of adverse effects of weight in patients with type 2 diabetes.

Aspirin

If you are at high risk of cardiovascular disease, then your doctor may suggest that you take aspirin every day. This is because aspirin thins the blood and makes it less likely that blood clots will form in your arteries, which have the potential to cause heart attacks and strokes. Many people are sensitive to aspirin and so you may be prescribed other 'blood-thinning' drugs such as clopidogrel (Plavix®) as an alternative.

For more information see
Type 2 diabetes

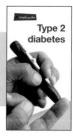

MANAGING MULTIPLE RISK FACTORS

You may worry that by being overweight and having multiple risk factors that you will end up taking loads of pills. In part this is true. Many obese people have to take five or more different drugs to manage all their different risk factors, plus other drugs for respiratory complications or for pain and discomfort. However, advances in drug technology mean that many of the drugs described in the earlier sections are available as a combination in a single tablet. In addition, many of the newer drugs that have been developed address many of the risk factors at the same time. For example, rimonabant has been shown not only to help you lose weight and reduce your waist size but can also improve other risk factors such as your lipid profile and your blood glucose level at the same time.

COMPLEMENTARY TREATMENTS

Complementary and alternative therapies may have some role in long-term weight control. However, they should not be considered as a replacement for the conventional approaches of lifestyle change and drug therapy as recommended by your doctor.

If you are taking a complementary or alternative treatment, you should always inform your doctor as some of these products may interfere with other drugs that he or she prescribes for you.

Complementary medicines generally lack the strong scientific evidence to back up claims regarding their effectiveness and safety. This is in contrast to licensed medicines that have to go through rigorous well-designed clinical trials performed in lots of people.

If you are considering using any herbal supplements to control your cholesterol, always consider the advice of the Medicines Control Agency:

- never buy herbal products abroad or by mail order

- only buy a herbal remedy if it states clearly which herbs it contains

- stop using herbal remedies if you experience any side-effects

- do not exceed the stated dose

- do not use if you are pregnant or breast-feeding.

COMPLEMENTARY MEDICINES WITH EVIDENCE FOR WEIGHT LOSS

Chitosan

Chitosan is a food supplement which contains a polysaccharide derived from shellfish like crabs and shrimps. It has similar properties to cellulose. Limited evidence suggests that chitosan given in conjunction with a calorie-controlled diet produces greater weight loss than diet alone. It may also reduce LDL-C and increase HDL-C.

Zotrim

Zotrim is a combination of three different herbs yerba maté, guarana and damiana. It works by slowing down the emptying of the stomach making you feel full more quickly and thus reducing the amount of food you eat. As you feel full for longer after eating, it may also reducing snacking between meals.

Hoodia cactus

Hoodia cactus has been used for many generations by the indigenous tribesmen of the Kalahari desert in Southern Africa as a natural appetite suppressant during long hunting trips. Hoodia works by mimicking biological processes that occur naturally after you eat. Glucose receptors in the hypothalamus of the brain recognise a chemical in hoodia cactus that is more potent than glucose itself at stimulating signals of fullness. As a consequence, you feel full even though you haven't eaten.

WHAT SHOULD I EXPECT FROM THE HEALTH SERVICE?

Obesity and overweight are frequently dismissed as a result of a series of poor lifestyle choices. Consequently, obese and overweight people often experience discrimination in their daily lives, even when they consult with their healthcare professionals. However, increasingly the healthcare community is accepting that obesity is a chronic disease in its own right and should be managed with empathy.

YOUR HEALTHCARE PROFESSIONAL TEAM

By working closely with your healthcare team and by being as honest and as open with them as possible you can expect to be more successful in your weight-loss programme.

You can expect to see a number of different healthcare professionals who have the responsibility of managing obesity and weight problems within your local community. The list below is a fairly complete list of the professionals that you or a member of your family may see during any weight-loss programme:

- GP
- practice nurse, school nurse and nurse specialist
- dietitian
- pharmacist
- exercise professional
- midwife
- health visitor
- specialists (such as a cardiologist or an endocrinologist).

PREVENTION OF OBESITY

If we are to have any impact on the long-term adverse effects of the current epidemic of obesity, we need to act now to address and reverse some of the changes in society that have created our 'obesogenic' environment.

A relatively small shift in the population's behaviour could radically improve the current situation. For example, small increases in the number of daily steps we take, small decreases in the amount of dietary fat and sugar we eat and smaller portion sizes could all have a positive impact on the current burden of obesity in the UK. In Finland, for example, public health campaigns and a programme of education that encouraged healthy eating led to a reduction in obesity by 25%. In the USA, it has been estimated that 90% of the obesity problem could be solved by everyone walking 2,000 more steps a day and by reducing daily energy intake by about 600 calories.

To encourage these changes requires a huge effort from, and co-operation between, government, schools, the food industry and food retailers, advertisers, architects and town planners. A number of strategies and policies may have an impact on the obesity problem, some of which have already been accepted by government.

■ Restrictions on TV advertising of unhealthy foods to children.

■ Clearer labelling of food to identify foods that are high in fat, sugar and salt.

■ 'Free fruit at school' schemes.

■ Restrictions on the sale of high-energy foods and drinks to children (e.g. banning fizzy drink and snack vending machines in schools).

■ Public health campaigns to promote healthier food choices (e.g. the 'five-a-day' campaign) and more active lifestyles.

■ A shift in transport policy away from cars and buses towards walking and cycling.

■ More opportunities for physical recreation.

Fizzy drinks are a particular problem. In the UK, more than 70% of children consume fizzy drinks on a regular basis. Schools and parents should encourage their children to drink more water and reduce the opportunities to buy these drinks. It has been estimated that by reducing fizzy drink consumption over 12 months in 7–11 year olds, we could reduce the prevalence of obesity and overweight by about 7.5%.

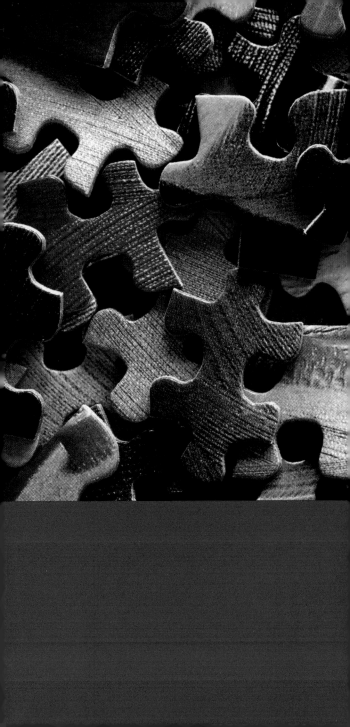